Patellofemoral Instability Decision Making and Techniques

Editor

DAVID R. DIDUCH

CLINICS IN SPORTS MEDICINE

www.sportsmed.theclinics.com

Consulting Editor
MARK D. MILLER

January 2022 • Volume 41 • Number 1

ELSEVIER

1600 John F. Kennedy Boulevard ● Suite 1800 ● Philadelphia, Pennsylvania, 19103-2899

http://www.theclinics.com

CLINICS IN SPORTS MEDICINE Volume 41, Number 1
January 2022 ISSN 0278-5919, ISBN-13: 978-0-323-84898-5

Editor: Lauren Boyle
Developmental Editor: Diana Grace Ang

Clinics in Sports Medicine (ISSN 0278-5919) is published quarterly by Elsevier Inc., 360 Park Avenue South, New York, NY 10010-1710. Months of issue are January, April, July, and October. Business and Editorial Offices: 1600 John F. Kennedy Blvd., Ste. 1800, Philadelphia, PA 19103-2899. Customer Service Office: 3251 Riverport Lane, Maryland Heights, MO 63043. Periodicals postage paid at New York, NY and additional mailing offices. Subscription prices are $368.00 per year (US individuals), $959.00 per year (US institutions), $100.00 per year (US students), $409.00 per year (Canadian individuals), $988.00 per year (Canadian institutions), $100.00 (Canadian students), $480.00 per year (foreign individuals), $988.00 per year (foreign institutions), and $235.00 per year (foreign students). Foreign air speed delivery is included in all *Clinics* subscription prices. All prices are subject to change without notice. **POSTMASTER:** Send address changes to *Clinics in Sports Medicine*, Elsevier Health Sciences Division, Subscription Customer Service, 3251 Riverport Lane, Maryland Heights, MO 63043. Customer Service (orders, claims, online, change of address): Elsevier Health Sciences Division, Subscription Customer Service, 3251 Riverport Lane, Maryland Heights, MO 63043. **Tel: 1-800-654-2452 (U.S. and Canada); 314-447-8871 (outside U.S. and Canada). Fax: 314-447-8029. E-mail: journalscustomerservice-usa@elsevier.com (for print support); journalsonlinesupport-usa@ elsevier.com (for online support).**

Reprints. For copies of 100 or more of articles in this publication, please contact the Commercial Reprints Department, Elsevier Inc., 360 Park Avenue South, New York, NY 10010-1710. Tel.: 212-633-3874; Fax: 212-633-3820; E-mail: reprints@elsevier.com.

Clinics in Sports Medicine is covered in *MEDLINE/PubMed (Index Medicus) Current Contents/Clinical Medicine, Excerpta Medica,* and *ISI/Biomed.*

Contributors

CONSULTING EDITOR

MARK D. MILLER, MD
S. Ward Casscells Professor, Department of Orthopaedic Surgery, University of Virginia, Charlottesville, Virginia, USA

EDITOR

DAVID R. DIDUCH, MD
Voshell Professor of Sports Medicine, Division Head, Sports Medicine, Head Orthopaedic Team Physician, Professor, Department of Orthopaedic Surgery, University of Virginia, Charlottesville, Virginia, USA

AUTHORS

MELISSA ALBERSHEIM, MD
Department of Orthopedic Surgery, University of Minnesota, Minneapolis, Minnesota, USA

GREGORY ANDERSON, MD
Fellow in Sports Medicine, Orthopaedic Surgery, University of Virginia, Charlottesville, Virginia, USA

ELIZABETH A. ARENDT, MD
Professor and Vice Chair, Department of Orthopedic Surgery, University of Minnesota, Minneapolis, Minnesota, USA

ROLAND M. BIEDERT, MD
Associate Professor of Orthopaedic Surgery and Sports Traumatology, SportsClinic#1, Bern, Switzerland

CAITLIN C. CHAMBERS, MD
Assistant Professor, Department of Orthopedic Surgery, University of Minnesota, Minneapolis, Minnesota, USA; TRIA Orthopedic Center, Woodbury, Minnesota, USA

MICHAEL CHAU, MD
Department of Orthopedic Surgery, University of Minnesota, Minneapolis, Minnesota, USA

TRENTON COOPER, DO
Gillette Children's Specialty Healthcare, St Paul, Minnesota, USA

ANDREW J. COSGAREA, MD
Drew Family Professor of Orthopaedic Surgery in Honor of Alec J Cosgarea, Department of Orthopaedic Surgery, The Johns Hopkins School of Medicine, Baltimore, Maryland, USA

NAVYA DANDU, BS
Rush University Medical Center, Chicago, Illinois, USA

REEM Y. DARWISH, BS
Rush University Medical Center, Chicago, Illinois, USA

STEVEN F. DEFRODA, MD
Rush University Medical Center, Chicago, Illinois, USA

DAVID H. DEJOUR, MD
Lyon-Ortho-Clinic, Clinique de la Sauvegarde, Ramsay Santé, Lyon, France

DAVID R. DIDUCH, MD
Voshell Professor of Sports Medicine, Division Head, Sports Medicine, Head Orthopaedic
Team Physician, Professor, Department of Orthopaedic Surgery, University of Virginia,
Charlottesville, Virginia, USA

JOHN P. FULKERSON, MD
Professor, Department of Orthopaedic Surgery and Rehabilitation, Yale University, Yale
School of Medicine, New Haven, Connecticut, USA

ELIZABETH C. GARDNER, MD
Associate Professor, Department of Orthopaedic Surgery and Rehabilitation, Yale
University, Yale School of Medicine, New Haven, Connecticut, USA

ALAN GETGOOD, MPhil MD FRCS(Tr&Orth)
Orthopaedic Surgeon, Assistant Professor, Fowler Kennedy Sports Medicine
Clinic/Department of Surgery, Western University, London, Ontario, Canada

EDOARDO GIOVANNETTI DE SANCTIS, MD
Lyon-Ortho-Clinic, Clinique de la Sauvegarde, Ramsay Santé, Lyon, France

ANDREAS H. GOMOLL, MD
Hospital for Special Surgery, New York, New York, USA

DANIEL W. GREEN, MD, MS, FACS
Department of Pediatric Orthopedics, Hospital for Special Surgery, New York, New York,
USA

PHILLIP T. GRISDELA, MD
Resident Physician, Department of Orthopaedic Surgery, Massachusetts General
Hospital, Harvard Medical School, Boston, Massachusetts, USA

BETINA B. HINCKEL, MD, PhD
Assistant Professor, Oakland University, Rochester, Michigan, USA; Department of
Orthopaedic Surgery, William Beaumont Hospital, Royal Oak, Michigan, USA

CHRISTOPHER M. LAPRADE, MD
Department of Orthopaedic Surgery, Stanford University, Stanford, California, USA

MARK T. LANGHANS, MD, PhD
Hospital for Special Surgery, New York, New York, USA

MICHAELA I. McCARTHY, MD
Department of Orthopedic Surgery, University of Minnesota, Minneapolis, Minnesota,
USA

GUILLAUME MESNARD, MD
Lyon-Ortho-Clinic, Clinique de la Sauvegarde, Ramsay Santé, Lyon, France

DAVID A. MOLHO, MD
Resident, Department of Orthopaedic Surgery and Rehabilitation, Yale University, Yale School of Medicine, New Haven, Connecticut, USA

IAIN R. MURRAY, MD, PhD
Department of Orthopaedic Surgery, Stanford University, Stanford, California, USA

BENJAMIN NOONAN, MD
Sanford Orthopedics & Sports Medicine, Fargo, North Dakota, USA

NIKOLAOS PASCHOS, MD, PhD
Instructor, Department of Orthopaedic Surgery, Massachusetts General Hospital, Harvard Medical School, Boston, Massachusetts, USA

SOFIA HIDALGO PEREA, BS
Department of Pediatric Orthopedics, Hospital for Special Surgery, New York, New York, USA

WILLIAM MICHAEL PULLEN, MD
Department of Orthopaedic Surgery, Stanford University, Stanford, California, USA

DAVIS L. ROGERS, MD
Department of Orthopaedic Surgery, The Johns Hopkins School of Medicine, Baltimore, Maryland, USA

SARA R. SHANNON
Department of Neuroscience, Duke University, Durham, North Carolina, USA

SETH L. SHERMAN, MD
Department of Orthopaedic Surgery, Stanford University, Stanford, California, USA

SABRINA M. STRICKLAND, MD
Hospital for Special Surgery, New York, New York, USA

MIHO J. TANAKA, MD
Member of the Faculty, Department of Orthopaedic Surgery, Massachusetts General Hospital, Harvard Medical School, Boston, Massachusetts, USA

SCOTT TAYLOR, MBBS(Hons), BMedSc, FRACS(Orth), FAOrthA
Clinical Fellow, Fowler Kennedy Sports Medicine Clinic/Department of Surgery, Western University, London, Ontario, Canada

MARC TOMPKINS, MD
Department of Orthopedic Surgery, University of Minnesota, Minneapolis, Minnesota, USA

NICHOLAS A. TRASOLINI, MD
Rush University Medical Center, Chicago, Illinois, USA

ADAM B. YANKE, MD, PhD
Rush University Medical Center, Chicago, Illinois, USA

Contents

> Patellofemoral pain is one of the most common symptoms of patients presenting to sports medicine clinics. Obtaining a pertinent history and performing a thorough examination is crucial to identifying the subset of patients with instability who are most likely to benefit from surgical stabilization. A comprehensive radiographic work-up that includes standard radiographs and advanced imaging helps elucidate the diagnosis and provides crucial information for preoperative planning. This article reviews the evaluation, physical examination, and interpretation of radiographic imaging of patients with patellofemoral pain as an introduction to subsequent articles in this issue discussing surgical interventions.

> Coronal malalignment of the patellofemoral joint may contribute to both instability as well as pain and joint overload. The use of distal realignment procedures has evolved to include uniplanar and multiplanar osteotomies, which allows patient-specific treatment. With a careful understanding of the complex pathoanatomy, including osseous, soft tissue, and dynamic muscular factors, an appropriately designed tibial tubercle osteotomy (TTO) is an invaluable tool for the orthopedic surgeon to improve joint biomechanics and off-load articular injuries. Current techniques have improved TTO surgery to limit complications and produce reliably good results.

> Rotational deformity is a less common cause of patellar instability than trochlear dysplasia and patella alta. In some cases, rotational deformity is the primary bony factor producing the instability and should be corrected surgically. More research is needed on what are normal values for femoral version and tibial torsion, as well as when the axial plane alignment needs to be corrected. Many tools can be used to evaluate the axial

plane and surgeons should be familiar with each of them. Understanding the advantages and disadvantages of each site for osteotomy will help the surgeon choose the most appropriate osteotomy.

Valgus malalignment is an important risk factor in recurrent patella instability. This article explores the role of corrective osteotomy and discusses the various described methods both on the femoral and tibial sides of the joint. A detailed operative technique of medial closing wedge distal femoral osteotomy is included.

Patella alta is described as abnormally high-riding patella in relation to the femur, the trochlear groove, or the tibia with decreased bony stability. Patella alta represents an important predisposing factor for patellofemoral instability. Different measurement methods are used to define patella alta. Despite the clinical importance of patella alta, there is only limited consensus on cutoff values, indications for treatment, and ideal correction. In addition, the impact of patella alta on other risk factors for lateral patellar instability is significant. This must be considered when assessing clinical complaints and choosing the best individual treatment. Combined surgical interventions may be necessary.

When? Only patients with high-grade trochlear dysplasia types B and D, in which the prominence of the trochlea (supratrochlear spur) is over 5 mm, recurrent patellar dislocation, and maltracking. How? Sulcus deepening trochleoplasty: modifies the trochlear shape with a central groove and oblique medial and lateral facets; decreases the patellofemoral joint reaction force by reducing the trochlear prominence (spur); and reduces the tibial tubercle and the trochlear groove value by a proximal realignment. Pros: This procedure is highly effective in restoring patellofemoral stability and satisfying the patients. Cons: The patients must be aware of the risk of continuing residual pain and range-ofmotion limitation and that the development of patellofemoral osteoarthritis is not predictable.

Medial patellofemoral ligament reconstruction is used increasingly to treat patellar instability. A number of different techniques have been described to perform this procedure. In this article, we review common pearls and pitfalls to medial patellofemoral ligament reconstruction, as well as tips for troubleshooting the procedure. A special emphasis is placed on femoral tunnel position and intraoperative adjustments that can be made to improve outcomes.

Through this article, the authors aim to summarize the techniques performed on both first time and recurrent skeletally immature patients experiencing patellar dislocation. This article focuses on several key points, such as the importance of medial patellofemoral ligament femoral insertions being distal to the growth plate and performing extensive lateral release and quadricep tendon lengthening in cases of obligatory dislocation. Although acknowledging the procedures discussed cannot be considered for all patients, as individuals with open growth plates may require additional operative time, in many cases these techniques yield high rates of success.

Management of the patient with multiple risk factors for recurrent patellar instability is complex. Surgeons must possess familiarity with the anatomic risk factors that are associated with first time and recurrent instability events and weigh them in the patient's individualized surgical "menu" options for surgical patellar stabilization. Addressing individual risk factors, pairing imaging findings with physical examination, and thoughts on prioritizing risk factors to determine which should be prioritized for surgical correction are discussed.

Congenital dislocation of the patella is a rare condition characterized by lateral dislocation of the patella that is irreducible without surgical correction. Although there is no clear inheritance pattern, it is associated with several congenital syndromes. Patients often demonstrate flexion contracture, loss of active knee extension, increased tibial external rotation, and absent patella in the trochlea. Treatment requires surgical management and is comprised of lateral release, medial stabilization, quadriceps lengthening, and distal realignment. Results are generally favorable after treatment; persistent flexion contracture and redislocation are the most common complications. Further study is needed to define the optimal timing and treatment strategy for this uncommon condition.

Cartilage defects of the patellofemoral joint are commonly found in association with patellar instability owing to abnormal biomechanics. Strategies to address chondral defects of the patellofemoral joint secondary to instability should first address causes of recurrent instability. Most patello-femoral chondral defects associated with instability are less than 2 cm2 and do not generally require intervention beyond chondroplasty. Larger defects of the patella and/or the trochlea can be repaired with osteochondral or surface cartilage repair.

Iain R. Murray, Christopher M. LaPrade, William Michael Pullen, and Seth L. Sherman

Patellar instability is one of the most prevalent knee disorders, with dislocations occurring in 5 to 43 cases per 10,000 annually. Traumatic patellar dislocation can result in significant morbidity and is associated with patellofemoral chondral injuries and fractures, medial soft tissue disruption, pain, and reduced function, and can lead to patellofemoral osteoarthritis. Chronic and recurrent instability can lead to deformation and incompetence of the medial soft tissue stabilizers. Despite recent gains in understanding the pathoanatomy of this disorder, the management of patients with this condition is complex and remains enigmatic.

Navya Dandu, Nicholas A. Trasolini, Steven F. DeFroda, Reem Y. Darwish, and Adam B. Yanke

The lateral patellofemoral complex is an important stabilizer to medial and lateral displacement of the patella. Soft tissue abnormalities can range from pathologic tightness to laxity, presenting with symptoms related to patellar instability, anterior knee pain, or arthritis. Clinical evaluation should be performed to confirm patellar dislocation, assess the integrity of the lateral and medial soft tissues, and explore other pathoanatomic factors that may need to be addressed. Lateral retinacular lengthening is recommended over lateral release owing to the potential of iatrogenic medial instability with release, and a lateral patellofemoral ligament reconstruction can be performed to effectively treat medial instability.

CLINICS IN SPORTS MEDICINE

FORTHCOMING ISSUES

April 2022
Sports Anesthesia
Ashley Shilling, *Editor*

July 2022
Sports Cardiology
Dean Nelson Peter, *Editor*

October 2022
Pediatric & Adolescent Knee Injuries:
Evaluation, Treatment & Rehabilitation
Matthew D. Milewski, *Editor*

RECENT ISSUES

October 2021
Sports Medicine Imaging
Nicholas C. Nacey, Jennifer L. Pierce,
Editors

July 2021
Sports Spine
Adam Shimer and Francis H. Shen, *Editors*

April 2021
Athletic Injuries of the Hip
Dustin L. Richter and F. Winston
Gwathmey, *Editors*

SERIES OF RELATED INTERESTED

Orthopedic Clinics
https://www.orthopedic.theclinics.com/
Foot and Ankle Clinics
https://www.foot.theclinics.com/
Hand Clinics
https://www.hand.theclinics.com/
Physical Medicine and Rehabilitation Clinics
https://www.pmr.theclinics.com/

THE CLINICS ARE AVAILABLE ONLINE!
Access your subscription at:
www.theclinics.com

Foreword

Patellar Instability—The Great Imitator

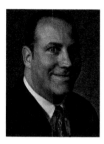

Mark D. Miller, MD
Consulting Editor

Many diseases in medicine have been dubbed "Great Imitators" to include syphilis and, more recently, Lyme disease. In the orthopedic world, patellar instability can be added to that list. I recently offered to see a young athlete who injured his knee. He was from the high school football team that my partner takes care of. He had an effusion and was difficult to examine, so I assumed that he had an ACL injury, sent the boy off for an MRI, and arranged for follow-up with him. I later learned that the player actually had a patellar dislocation and had a TT-TG measurement of 25 mm. Ironically, that partner is an international expert in patellofemoral instability and the Guest Editor of this issue of *Clinics in Sports Medicine*. So, despite my embarrassment, at least this young man ended up with the right surgeon. Unfortunately, this was not the first time that I have made this mistake, and many of you, if you are honest, have done the same thing. Acute patella dislocations often present just like acute ACL tears and have hence been added to the "Great Imitator" list.

This issue of *Clinics in Sports Medicine* is an international treatise on the management of patellar instability. It includes all directions, all components, all ages, and all variants. I am a huge fan of the article in this issue entitled, "Putting it all Together: Evaluating Patella Instability Risk Factors: Revisiting the 'Menu,' " by McCarthy and colleagues that puts it all together. If you have time to read just one article in this issue, focus on that one. My sincere appreciation to my partner and editor for this issue, Dr

Clin Sports Med 41 (2022) xiii–xiv
https://doi.org/10.1016/j.csm.2021.09.002
0278-5919/22/© 2021 Published by Elsevier Inc.

David Diduch, who has climbed the ladder of the patellofemoral world experts and has "capped" his career in this area.

Mark D. Miller, MD
Division of Sports Medicine
Department of Orthopaedic Surgery
University of Virginia, Charlottesville
400 Ray C. Hunt Drive, Suite 330
Charlottesville, VA 22908-0159, USA

E-mail address:
MDM3P@hscmail.mcc.virginia.edu

Preface

There Is a Lot Going on with that Knee....

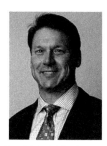

David R. Diduch, MD
Editor

So often, as we evaluate patients with patella instability, this is the phrase I hear from residents, fellows, and colleagues. There are numerous anatomic risk factors in play, often with several at once. Which are important? Which meet a threshold value to consider correction? Which combinations are most problematic? And how do the "experts" correct the anatomy? Decision making in this arena is critical—probably as much as technique.

This publication provides the framework to evaluate a patient with patellar instability and accurately quantify the forces at work to create recurrent dislocations. Experts from across the world have contributed articles outlining how they approach these various anatomic risk factors and techniques to correct the anatomy. Plus, more importantly, guidance on when to correct them. Coronal malalignment, rotational deformity, valgus alignment, patella alta, and trochlear dysplasia are all covered. Plus, an article on how to put it all together. These are the "thought leaders" in the patellofemoral world sharing their wisdom and expertise, from the basic to the most difficult. We also provide the framework for doing an medial patellofemoral ligament (MPFL) reconstruction well, and how to manage open growth plates. When and how should the surgeon address the lateral retinaculum, whether tight or iatrogenically loose? And what about the congenital, fixed lateral dislocation, and how to best manage associated chondral defects.

Clin Sports Med 41 (2022) xv–xvi
https://doi.org/10.1016/j.csm.2021.09.003
0278-5919/22/© 2021 Published by Elsevier Inc.

sportsmed.theclinics.com

This resource covers the entire spectrum that a surgeon will encounter treating patellar instability patients. We hope you will find the tools you need to develop a solid plan to help your patients.

David R. Diduch, MD
Department of Orthopaedic Surgery
University of Virginia
Charlottesville, VA 22903, USA

E-mail address:
drd5c@virginia.edu

Evaluating Patellofemoral Patients

Physical Examination, Radiographic Imaging, and Measurements

Davis L. Rogers, MD, Andrew J. Cosgarea, MD*

KEYWORDS

- Patella dislocation • Patella instability • Patellofemoral pain • Malalignment
- Maltracking

KEY POINTS

- Patellofemoral disorders are among the most common diagnoses of patients presenting to sports medicine physicians.
- Key contributors to patellofemoral pain include biologic and mechanical factors.
- It is crucial to identify patellofemoral patients with instability because surgical intervention can mitigate functional deficits and prevent recurrence.
- The diagnosis of recurrent patellar dislocation is typically straightforward, whereas subtle subluxation episodes are more difficult to identify.
- Clinical findings of malalignment and maltracking during physical examination suggest a predisposition to instability; provocative maneuvers can confirm the diagnosis.
- Radiographs and advanced imaging are used to identify anatomic and morphologic abnormities to confirm the diagnosis and provide key information for surgical planning.

INTRODUCTION
Background

Nearly one-third of all knee pain is related to the patellofemoral joint.[1] The diagnosis of "patellofemoral pain" simply refers to the anatomic location from where the pain arises. Often previously called "chondromalacia patellae," or "anterior knee pain," patellofemoral pain has a variety of causes. The most common causes relate to articular surface overload and instability, but the cause in any given patient is often multi-factorial. Patellofemoral pain syndrome is a nonspecific diagnosis used to describe patients who have no demonstrable anatomic lesion. Patients typically describe

Department of Orthopaedic Surgery, Johns Hopkins Outpatient Center, 601 North Caroline Street, 5th Floor, Baltimore, MD 21287, USA
* Corresponding author.
E-mail address: acosgar@jhmi.edu

Clin Sports Med 41 (2022) 1–13
https://doi.org/10.1016/j.csm.2021.07.001
0278-5919/22/© 2021 Elsevier Inc. All rights reserved.

retropatellar pain that is exacerbated by stair climbing or descending, prolonged sitting, and running. It is typically a diagnosis of exclusion.

Patients with patellar instability make up a small subset of patients presenting with patellofemoral pain. They experience specific episodes that often interfere with job responsibilities and recreational activities. Patients with frank dislocation typically describe painful episodes where the patella dramatically displaces and may spontaneously reduce or require a manual reduction. Less obvious, however, is the history of subluxation, which is subtle, causing symptoms ranging from transient discomfort to substantial functional instability. Identification of patients with instability is crucial because successful surgical intervention can minimize disability and decrease the likelihood of progressive joint destruction, which is caused by recurrent instability episodes. In this article, we describe the clinical and radiographic work-up for patients with patellofemoral pain to identify the patients with instability who could most benefit from surgical intervention.

Primary patellar dislocation has an estimated incidence of 5.8 per 100,000 persons,[2] a substantial portion of whom experience dislocation during the second or third decade of life.[3] The incidence of recurrent instability after a primary dislocation is estimated to be 15% to 44%.[4,5] The risk of recurrent instability is related to numerous physiologic and anatomic factors. In one study, the authors developed a "patellar instability severity" score[6] using six patient factors (age, presence of bilateral instability, patella alta, tibial tuberosity–trochlear groove [TT-TG] distance, patellar tilt, and trochlear dysplasia). They demonstrated a five-fold increase in the risk of recurrent patellar instability in patients who scored four or more compared with those who scored less than four. Other researchers described the "recurrent instability of the patella" score,[7] which uses four factors (skeletal maturity, age, trochlear dysplasia, and the ratio of TT-TG to patellar length) to identify patients as being at low, intermediate, or high risk for recurrence. These and a similar[8] study demonstrate the importance of identifying anatomic and physiologic risk factors to estimate risk of recurrence and provide patients with appropriate treatment recommendations.

Patients with patellar instability can present many different ways, so it is important to understand relevant terminology. "Dislocation" indicates full displacement from the TG; patients typically report a painful sensation of dislocation or lateral patella shifting.[9] "Subluxation" is partial displacement of the patella out of the TG without definitive dislocation.[3] "Maltracking" describes deviation of the patella from the TG during the flexion-extension arc. Although subluxation and frank dislocation episodes are typically painful, patients with maltracking may be asymptomatic. "Laxity" refers to the amount of translation of the patella within the TG, which is quantified in quadrants. In contrast to laxity, the word "instability" suggests symptomatic pathologic laxity.

Anatomic Considerations

Knee pain is ultimately related to joint overload that typically results from anatomic or mechanical dysfunction. Patellar instability is caused by an imbalance between the numerous forces acting across the patellofemoral joint. The stability of the patella depends on three key factors: (1) dynamic muscle action, (2) osteochondral geometry, and (3) passive soft tissue restraints. The quadriceps muscles, and particularly the vastus medialis obliquus, dynamically stabilize the patellofemoral joint.[10] Weakness or deficiency of the vastus medialis obliquus, and core musculature and hip external rotators, is also believed to predispose to patellofemoral pain and instability.

The medial patellofemoral complex provides the primary soft tissue restraint to pathologic lateral translation of the patella. The most important component of the medial patellofemoral complex is the medial patellofemoral ligament (MPFL). Other contributors include the medial patellomeniscal ligament, medial patellotibial ligament, and medial quadriceps tendon femoral ligament. The MPFL is most important biomechanically in the first 30° of knee flexion[11] and becomes less important with greater degrees of flexion.

Beyond 45° of knee flexion, the osteochondral geometry of the patellofemoral joint plays an increasingly important role in patellar stability.[10,12,13] If the lateral trochlear ridge is deficient, or the normally concave TG has a convex shape, as in the case of trochlear dysplasia, the patellofemoral joint loses an important component of its inherent anatomic stability. The term "malalignment" is used to describe abnormal skeletal alignment. Malalignment contributes to an imbalance in the factors that normally stabilize the patella by altering muscle forces and undermining normal structural integrity.[14] Malalignment is seen in the axial plane as excessive femoral anteversion or tibial torsion, both of which increase laterally directed forces on the patella. Trochlear dysplasia and patella alta are seen in the sagittal plane; patella alta exacerbates the structural deficiencies caused by trochlear dysplasia. With patella alta, the knee must flex to a greater degree before the patella engages in the TG, increasing the risk of dislocation. Excessive valgus alignment and lateralized TT are both examples of malalignment in the coronal plane.

CLINICAL EVALUATION
History of Presentation

Age and female sex are known risk factors for causes of patellofemoral pain (eg, patients younger than 16 years have a greater risk of recurrent instability).[6] Along with age, skeletal maturity may influence the choice of treatment.[7,15]

When asking about patellofemoral symptoms, it is important to ascertain specific location, inciting factors, and exacerbating activities. Patients with patellofemoral pain frequently report pain with standing from sitting, traversing stairs, or other activities involving knee flexion. Many patients with instability describe episodes of lateral displacement, followed by spontaneous or manual reduction of the patella. Ask about the contralateral knee because risk factors for malalignment frequently occur bilaterally. Patients who report an episode of instability are three times as likely to experience a contralateral dislocation compared with the general population.[16] Descriptive features of the pain help: constant pain may be radicular or referred; sharp intermittent pain unrelated to specific activity may suggest a loose body, unstable cartilage, or impending tissue compression; activity-related pain likely reflects joint overload, maltracking of the patellofemoral joint, or inflammatory conditions of the knee.

Note previous treatment, including physical therapy or bracing, and the frequency and duration of pain medication use. Ask about comorbidities, particularly obesity, diabetes, inflammatory arthropathies, rheumatologic conditions, and recent or chronic use of steroids.

Physical Examination

Assess patient comfort level; be aware of the patient's level of anxiety, which may affect their ability to relax and undermine the physician's ability to interpret the examination. Visualize gait to identify an antalgic pattern. Specifically, look for signs of quadriceps or hip abductor weakness. Core strength is assessed by asking the patient to perform a single-leg squat. Assess standing alignment for obvious varus or valgus deformity or leg-length discrepancy. Examine the contralateral extremity first because it provides a baseline comparison and gives the patient a sense of what to expect for the symptomatic extremity. Follow a standard physical examination routine so no important aspects are overlooked.

Inspect the extremity for abrasions, swelling, bruising, and muscle atrophy. Patients with a substantial effusion can appear to lose normal surface contour. The medial gutter may have a convex appearance rather than the normal concave shape. "Milking" the medial gutter, followed by applying pressure on the lateral gutter, can demonstrate a fluid wave, confirming the presence of a clinically relevant effusion. Even a small effusion can produce quadriceps inhibition and/or weakness.[17]

Palpate the components of the extensor mechanism that could be contributing to the patient's pain, including the quadriceps tendon, patella, patellar tendon, and TT. Continue with palpation of the medial and lateral sides of the knee, including the joint lines and collateral ligaments. It is not unusual to sustain a medial collateral ligament injury at the time of patellar dislocation. Patients who have sustained a recent dislocation often report tenderness along the course of the MPFL, between its attachment on the medial border of the patella and the femoral insertion site between the adductor tubercle and medial epicondyle.

Perform a standard neurovascular and ligamentous knee examination to rule out more serious pathology. Document range of motion, including hyperextension. Joint hyperlaxity, a known risk factor for instability, is quantified with the Beighton hypermobility score.[18] In addition to knee hyperextension, this score incorporates thumb, little finger, elbow, and trunk range of motion to help define criteria for hypermobility syndrome. Assess quadriceps tightness by measuring the distance from the heel to the buttock with the patient prone. Calf, hamstring, and iliotibial band tightness should be checked. The patellar tilt test is performed by manually elevating the lateral portion of the patella. Inability to elevate the lateral patella past horizontal suggests a tight lateral retinaculum. Patellar glide, assessed by measuring the amount of patellar translation after applying a medial or lateral force, provides information about the integrity of soft tissue restraints. The distance of translation is quantified in patella width quadrants, with one quadrant representing approximately 10 mm in the typical patella (**Fig. 1**). Compare laxity with that of the contralateral side.

Patellofemoral function is affected by alignment of the entire limb; thus, evaluation is not limited to the knee. Excessive femoral anteversion and tibial torsion are risk factors for lateral patellar instability. Femoral anteversion is assessed with the patient prone; excessive anteversion is defined by internal rotation of the hip exceeding that of external rotation.[3] Tibial torsion is assessed by visualizing the apparent angle between the transepicondylar femoral axis and the transmalleolar tibial axis.[3] Some clinicians measure the Q-angle, formed by lines drawn from the center of the patella to the anterior superior iliac spine and to the TT.[19] Although this represents an approximation of the overall lateral force vector on the patella, an increased Q-angle may be caused by excessive valgus alignment, lateralized TT, or both. The usefulness of this measurement is limited by inconsistency in reproducibility.[3]

The J-sign is a dynamic manifestation of patellar maltracking,[20] representing the sum of all active and passive forces acting on the patellofemoral joint. The seated patient is asked to actively extend the knee against gravity as the physician observes the trajectory of the patella. Deviation of normal midline tracking of the patella, particularly in terminal extension, is called a J-sign (**Fig. 2**). Other maltracking patterns have also been described, including dislocation in flexion. In a recent study of the reliability of visual assessment of patellar tracking, the authors reported that 68% of surgeons could identify the presence of maltracking, whereas only half could accurately specify the grade.[21] As with most physical examination tests, positive findings do not necessarily imply functional instability. The presence of maltracking and hyperlaxity helps

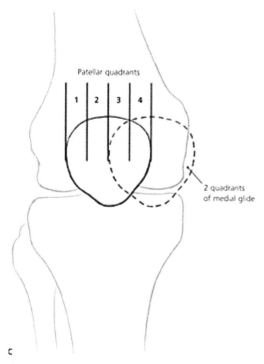

Fig. 1. Illustration of the patellar glide test, which is performed medially (as depicted) or laterally. (*Reprinted* with permission from Todd Buck, medical illustrator of Figure 2 in: Dixit S, DiFiori JP, Burton M, et al. Management of patellofemoral pain syndrome. Am Fam Physician. 2007;75(2):194-202. © 2007 Todd Buc.)

confirm the diagnosis and provides the surgeon with information on how to treat the instability.

Provocative tests are typically reserved for the end of the physical examination because they are the most likely to be uncomfortable. The patellar grind test is performed by asking the patient to activate the quadriceps while the examiner manually loads the patella. Crepitus may be felt or heard. Perform the patellar apprehension test[22] by manually translating the patella laterally and asking if this makes the patient apprehensive or reproduces their sensation of instability. The medial patellar apprehension test involves translating the patella medially while simultaneously flexing the knee. Although uncommon, medial instability is suggested if this test reproduces the patient's sensation, especially in patients who have undergone lateral retinacular release.

Radiographic Imaging

Initial radiographic work-up should include anteroposterior (AP), lateral, notch, and axial views.[23] The lateral view, performed in 30° of knee flexion with superimposed medial and lateral femoral condyles, is used to diagnose patella alta, trochlear dysplasia,[24] and arthrosis.[25] More than 25% of patients who have had patellar dislocations have radiographic evidence of patella alta.[26] Traditionally, the Insall-Salvati[27] method was used to calculate patellar height. The Caton-Deschamps index is now the preferred method because it reflects changes in patellar position after TT distalization.

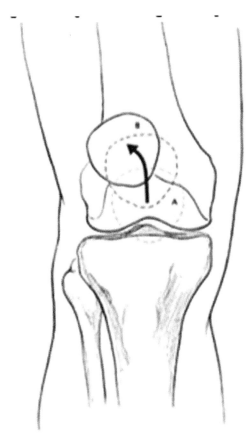

Fig. 2. Illustration of lateral patellar trajectory, or J-sign, during knee extension. The *dotted lines* encompassing A represent the initial location of the patella in the trochlear groove in knee flexion. B represents a laterally displaced patella as the patella moves superiorly out of the trochlear groove in knee extension. (*Reprinted* with permission from Todd Buck, medical illustrator of Figure 2 in: Dixit S, DiFiori JP, Burton M, et al. Management of patellofemoral pain syndrome. Am Fam Physician. 2007;75(2):194-202. © 2007 Todd Buc.)

The Caton-Deschamps index is calculated as the ratio between the distance from the inferior-most point of the patella articular cartilage to the anterior-most projection of the tibial plateau and the patellar articular length, with most clinicians considering a normal value to be less than or equal to 1.2 (**Fig. 3**).[10] The lateral view is also used to identify and classify trochlear dysplasia via the Dejour classification.[26] Type A trochlear dysplasia is identified by the crossing sign, when the cortices of the trochlear floor and lateral femoral condyle intersect, or cross; type B has a crossing sign in the presence of a trochlear spur; type C has a crossing sign and a double contour sign, where the anterior cortices of a substantially smaller medial femoral condyle become evident; and type D has a crossing sign, trochlear spur, and double contour sign (a combination of types A, B, and C) (**Fig. 4**). Up to 85% of patients with recurrent instability have some degree of trochlear dysplasia.[26]

Axial, or "sunrise," views are particularly useful in identifying dysplasia, arthrosis,[28] malalignment,[24] subluxation,[29] and tilt.[25,30] The merchant view is an axial view performed with the patient supine, the knee flexed to 45°, and the radiograph projected

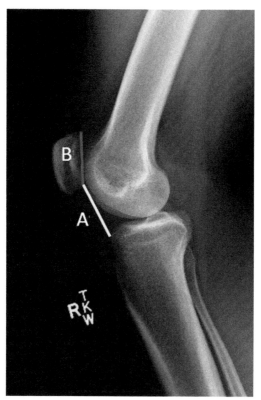

Fig. 3. Lateral radiograph showing measurement of Caton-Deschamps index, calculated as the ratio of the distance A, measured from the inferior-most point of the patellar articular surface to the anterior-most point of the tibial plateau, divided by B, the length of the patellar articular surface. Patella alta is defined as Caton-Deschamps index greater than 1.2.

inferiorly at 30° relative to the femur.[29] Normative data have been published for specific measurements taken from the merchant view. The sulcus angle[31] is formed between tangential lines along the medial and lateral trochlear ridges meeting at the deepest point in the TG. An angle greater than 145° is abnormal, suggesting a flat trochlea. The congruence angle[31] is formed by a line bisecting the sulcus angle and a line through the deepest portion of the patella. This measure indicates how well the patella is centered in the TG, with values less than 16° considered normal. The lateral patellofemoral angle[31] is calculated as the angle between a line along the lateral patellar facet and a line connecting the anterior-most portions of the trochlear ridges. In 97% of healthy knees, this angle opens laterally. Axial views are incorporated into the classification scheme used by Dejour and colleagues[26] to describe trochlear dysplasia.

AP views show arthrosis and tibiofemoral alignment. If there is concern for excessive malalignment in the coronal plane, standing long-leg AP radiographs may be obtained.[15] Notch views, performed with the knee in 40° of flexion, are useful for suspected occult osteochondritis dissecans lesions of the femoral condyles or loose bodies.[31] The posteroanterior weight-bearing 45°-flexion view (ie, Rosenberg view) is recommended for older patients or patients in whom subtle arthrosis is suspected.[15]

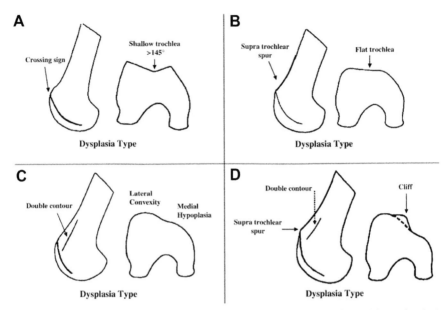

Fig. 4. Schematic drawings showing the Dejour classification of trochlear dysplasia, increasing in severity from type A to type D. (*A*) Crossing sign seen in the superior trochlea, suggesting a shallow trochlea. (*B*) Supratrochlear spur in the setting of a crossing sign, suggesting a flattened trochlea. (*C*) Crossing sign, and a double contour sign, suggesting a hypoplastic medial femoral condyle. (*D*) Combination of all three, in which the crossing sign, double contour sign, and supratrochlear spur are visualized. (Figure 4 reprinted with permission from Dejour D, Le Coultre B. Osteotomies in Patello-Femoral Instabilities. Sports Med Arthrosc Rev. 2007 Mar; 15(1):39-46. **Figure 2**)

Advanced Imaging

Advanced imaging offers advantages over conventional radiographs. MRI provides valuable information regarding articular cartilage, soft tissue damage,[32] and the presence of loose bodies,[15] particularly if acute episodes of instability or ligamentous damage are suspected. In the setting of a recent dislocation, MRI may show classic cartilage damage or bone bruising patterns involving the medial facet of the patella and lateral femoral condyle.[33,34] MRI is 85% sensitive and 70% accurate in detecting an acute injury of the MPFL.[35] It may also show proximal migration of, or edema over, the vastus medialis oblique, which can accompany MPFL injuries.[35] Computed tomography (CT) helps assess patellofemoral morphology, axial alignment, and arthrosis and is particularly useful for preoperative planning. When analyzing axial alignment, it is more efficient and economical to obtain CT scans of the entire lower extremity compared with the numerous MRI scans that would be necessary. However, the benefits of this approach should be weighed against the modest radiation exposure.[36] The greatest advantage of advanced imaging over conventional radiographs is the ability to perform measurements with accuracy. CT and MRI images can be reconstructed in any plane to optimize accuracy and reliability of measurements.[25,37] Accurate measurement of pathoanatomy allows the clinician to plan a surgical procedure to correct the abnormality contributing to instability episodes.

In the coronal plan, the greatest risk factor for recurrent instability is a lateralized TT. Lateralization of the tuberosity is quantified by measuring TT-TG distance.[38] This measure is the distance between two lines drawn perpendicular to a posterior condylar reference line, which pass through the extensor mechanism insertion point and the deepest portion of the TG.[39] The insertion point of the extensor mechanism is considered the center of the TT on CT and the distal insertion of the patellar tendon on MRI.[40] Most clinicians believe that normal TT-TG distance measured by CT scan is up to 15 to 20 mm.[26] The normal TT-TG distance measured by MRI is 2.3-3.8 mm[41] greater than when measured by CT.[42] TT-TG distance measurement is more difficult in the setting of trochlear dysplasia, because identification of the TG reference point has been found to be highly examiner-dependent.[43] When using this measure as a threshold to make surgical decisions, it is important to understand how imaging conditions, such as weight-bearing, changes in knee flexion angle, and active quadriceps contraction, affect TT-TG measurements.[44] As an alternative to TT-TG, the TT-to-posterior cruciate ligament (TT-PCL) distance can be measured on MRI. TT-PCL is measured identically to TT-TG, except the medial-most attachment of the PCL on the tibia is used instead of the TG.[40] TT-PCL measurements greater than 24 mm are considered abnormal.[42] Inherent in the use of the TT-TG and TT-PCL measurements is the limitation that these are absolute values that do not take into consideration the patient's height.

Patella alta and trochlear dysplasia are risk factors for recurrent instability in the sagittal plane.[6] Sagittal engagement is calculated through the patellotrochlear index: the ratio of trochlear to patellar articular cartilage on a sagittal MRI slice at the midline of the knee.[45] This measurement is an accurate reflection of the functional height of the patella. A patellotrochlear index of less than 12.5% suggests an abnormally proximal patella (patella alta) or an abnormally distal trochlea, both of which predispose to instability.[45] Understanding the relationship of the patella to the TG is crucial for surgeons considering a tibial tubercle distalizing osteotomy. CT and MRI greatly improve the appreciation of the complex morphology associated with trochlear dysplasia. These imaging modalities also allow accurate measurements of the trochlear bump, the magnitude of which many consider an indication for trochleoplasty.

MRI and CT are particularly valuable in providing accurate measurements of axial alignment and trochlear morphology. Femoral anteversion is measured using superimposed axial CT images of the proximal and distal femur, and tibial torsion is measured similarly by using superimposed images of the proximal and distal tibia. Derotational

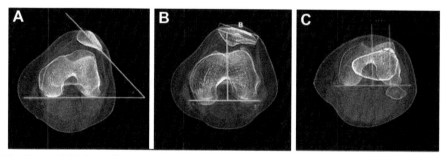

Fig. 5. Axial CT views demonstrating measurements of patellar tilt, bisect offset, and TT-TG distance. (A) Patellar tilt is the angle of tilt of the patella relative to the posterior femoral condyles, where normal is less than 15°. (B) Bisect offset is the percentage of the patella width lateral to the trochlear groove, in which normal is less than 66%. (C) TT-TG distance measures the lateralization of the tibial tuberosity relative to the trochlear groove, in which normal is up to 15-20 mm.

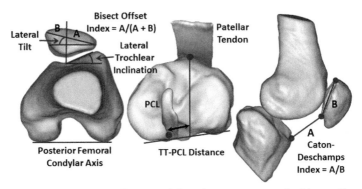

Fig. 6. Examples of reconstructed knee models with measurements for bisect offset, patellar tilt, trochlear inclination, TT-PCL distance, and Caton-Deschamps index. (Figure 6 reprinted from: Conry KT, Cosgarea AJ, Tanaka MJ, Elias JJ: Influence of Tibial Tuberosity Position and Trochlear Depth on Patellar Tracking in Patellar Instability: Variations with Patella Alta. Clinical Biomechanics. Under revision, 2021.)

osteotomies may be considered in cases of axial malrotation. Lateral patellar tilt is the angle formed between a line drawn across the posterior condyles and the midpatellar line, with angles greater than 15° suggestive of lateral retinacular tightness.[24] Bisect offset is calculated as the percentage of the patella that lies lateral to the femoral midline, in which less than 66% is considered normal (**Fig. 5**).[46] Measuring the depth of the TG on axial cuts helps to characterize the degree of trochlear dysplasia.[24] Trochlear inclination, the angle between a posterior condyle reference line and the lateral trochlear wall, suggests a deficient lateral trochlear ridge and is abnormal when less than 11° (**Fig. 6**).[24]

Dynamic CT and MRI are powerful imaging modalities performed while a patient actively moves the knee. Muscle activation enables a more functionally relevant analysis of tracking,[36] providing an understanding of patellar function that is unavailable from conventional radiographs and static CT and MRI studies. Accurate measurements of the bisect offset during active knee extension allow more accurate quantification of patellar maltracking than the visual assessment of the J-sign during clinical examination.[21] The imaging data can also be used to create computational models that can provide valuable information for surgical planning. Currently, these dynamic imaging modalities are available at several academic hospitals.

SUMMARY

Evaluation of the patient with patellofemoral pain requires a thorough understanding of the pertinent aspects of the history and physical examination. Identifying patients with recurrent patellar instability using provocative clinical tests is crucial, because they are the most likely to benefit from surgical intervention. A thorough radiographic work-up helps identify patients with large loose bodies or intra-articular fractures that require acute surgical intervention. Identifying patella alta and trochlear dysplasia on radiographs helps the surgeon plan for patellar stabilization surgery. MRI provides valuable information regarding soft tissue and chondral pathology and can confirm the diagnosis of instability if the clinical picture is unclear. CT scans provide accurate and objective measurements regarding malalignment in the coronal plane as well as trochlear morphology. Dynamic CT and MRI can help the clinician and researcher better understand maltracking patterns. After all of this information is gathered and synthesized, the surgeon can present treatment options that best address the patient's functional instability.

CLINICS CARE POINTS

- Patellofemoral pain is a nonspecific diagnosis, identifying the etiology is critical to providing optimum care.
- Stability of the patellofemoral joint depends on the contributions of dynamic muscle action, osteochondral geometry, and soft tissue restraints.
- Age, sex, skeletal maturity, and various anatomical variants are risk all factors for developing instability.
- Physical examination should include a thorough assessment of skeletal alignment and dynamic patellar tracking.
- Provocative tests such as the patellar apprehension sign are used to confirm the diagnosis of patellar instability.
- A complete set of radiographs is necessary to identify acute pathology like loose bodies and characterize bony malalignment.
- Advanced imaging allows for precise anatomical measurements of pathoanatomy to optimize preoperative planning.

DISCLOSURES

DLR has no conflicts to disclose. AJC is a member of the Board of Directors of the Patellofemoral Foundation and receives textbook royalties from Elsevier, Inc.

REFERENCES

1. Smith BE, Selfe J, Thacker D, et al. Incidence and prevalence of patellofemoral pain: a systematic review and meta-analysis. PLoS One 2018;13(1):e0190892.
2. Fithian DC, Paxton EW, Stone ML, et al. Epidemiology and natural history of acute patellar dislocation. Am J Sports Med 2004;32(5):1114–21.
3. Lattermann C, Arendt EA, Andrish J. Extensor mechanism injuries. In: Boyer MI, editor. AAOS comprehensive orthopaedic review. 2rd edition. Rosemont, IL: American Academy of Orthopaedic Surgeons; 2014. p. 1367–78.
4. Christensen TC, Sanders TL, Pareek A, et al. Risk factors and time to recurrent ipsilateral and contralateral patellar dislocations. Am J Sports Med 2017;45(9): 2105–10.
5. Lewallen L, McIntosh A, Dahm D. First-time patellofemoral dislocation: risk factors for recurrent instability. J knee Surg 2015;28(4):303–9.
6. Balcarek P, Oberthür S, Hopfensitz S, et al. Which patellae are likely to redislocate? Knee Surg Sports Traumatol Arthrosc 2014;22(10):2308–14.
7. Hevesi M, Heidenreich MJ, Camp CL, et al. The recurrent instability of the patella score: a statistically based model for prediction of long-term recurrence risk after first-time dislocation. Arthroscopy 2019;35(2):537–43.
8. Dixit S, DiFiori JP, Burton M, et al. Management of patellofemoral pain syndrome. Am Fam Physician 2007;75(2):194–202.
9. Post WR. Anterior knee pain: diagnosis and treatment. J Am Acad Orthop Surg 2005;13(8):534–43.

10. Tanaka MJ, Elias JJ, Cosgarea AJ. Patellofemoral joint disorders. In: Miller MD, editor. Orthopaedic knowledge update: sports medicine. 5th edition. Rosemont, IL: American Academy of Orthopaedic Surgeons; 2016. p. 205–19.

11. Desio SM, Burks RT, Bachus KN. Soft tissue restraints to lateral patellar translation in the human knee. Am J Sports Med 1998;26(1):59–65.

12. Diederichs G, Kohlitz T, Kornaropoulos E, et al. Magnetic resonance imaging analysis of rotational alignment in patients with patellar dislocations. Am J Sports Med 2013;41(1):51–7.

13. Latt LD, Christopher M, Nicolini A, et al. A validated cadaveric model of trochlear dysplasia. Knee Surg Sports Traumatol Arthrosc 2014;22(10):2357–63.

14. James SL, Bates BT, Osternig LR. Injuries to runners. Am J Sports Med 1978;6(2): 40–50.

15. Weber AE, Nathani A, Dines JS, et al. An algorithmic approach to the management of recurrent lateral patellar dislocation. J Bone Joint Surg Am 2016;98(5): 417–27.

16. Jaquith BP, Parikh SN. Predictors of recurrent patellar instability in children and adolescents after first-time dislocation. J Pediatr Orthop 2015;37(7):484–90.

17. Rice DA, McNair PJ, Lewis GN, et al. Quadriceps arthrogenic muscle inhibition: the effects of experimental knee joint effusion on motor cortex excitability. Arthritis Res Ther 2014;16(6):502.

18. Beighton P, Solomon L, Soskolne CL. Articular mobility in an African population. Ann Rheum Dis 1973;32(5):413–8.

19. Merchant AC, Fraiser R, Dragoo J, et al. A reliable Q angle measurement using a standardized protocol. Knee 2020;27(3):934–9.

20. Post WR. Clinical evaluation of patients with patellofemoral disorders. Arthroscopy 1999;15(8):841–51.

21. Best MJ, Tanaka MJ, Demehri S, et al. Accuracy and reliability of the visual assessment of patellar tracking. Am J Sports Med 2020;48(2):370–5.

22. Ahmad CS, McCarthy M, Gomez JA, et al. The moving patellar apprehension test for lateral patellar instability. Am J Sports Med 2009;37(4):791–6.

23. White BJ, Sherman OH. Patellofemoral instability. Bull NYU Hosp Jt Dis 2009; 67(1):22–9.

24. Haj-Mirzaian A, Thawait GK, Tanaka MJ, et al. Diagnosis and characterization of patellofemoral instability: review of available imaging modalities. Sports Med Arthrosc Rev 2017;25(2):64–71.

25. Merchant AC. Patellofemoral imaging. Clin Orthop 2001;389:15–21.

26. Dejour H, Walch G, Nove-Josserand L, et al. Factors of patellar instability: an anatomic radiographic study. Knee Surg Sports Traumatol Arthrosc 1994;2(1): 19–26.

27. Insall J, Salvati E. Patella position in the normal knee joint. Radiology 1971;101(1): 101–4.

28. Jungmann PM, Tham SC, Liebl H, et al. Association of trochlear dysplasia with degenerative abnormalities in the knee: data from the osteoarthritis initiative. Skeletal Radiol 2013;42(10):1383–92.

29. Merchant AC, Mercer RL, Jacobsen RH, et al. Roentgenographic analysis of patellofemoral congruence. J Bone Joint Surg Am 1974;56(7):1391–6.

30. Fulkerson JP. Patellofemoral pain disorders: evaluation and management. J Am Acad Orthop Surg 1994;2(2):124–32.

31. Endo Y, Shubin Stein BE, Potter HG. Radiologic assessment of patellofemoral pain in the athlete. Sports Health 2011;3(2):195–210.

32. Smith TO, Davies L, Toms AP, et al. The reliability and validity of radiological assessment for patellar instability. A systematic review and meta-analysis. Skeletal Radiol 2011;40(4):399–414.
33. Kirsch MD, Fitzgerald SW, Friedman H, et al. Transient lateral patellar dislocation: diagnosis with MR imaging. AJR Am J Roentgenol 1993;161(1):109–13.
34. Seeley MA, Knesek M, Vanderhave KL. Osteochondral injury after acute patellar dislocation in children and adolescents. J Pediatr Orthop 2013;33(5):511–8.
35. Sanders TG, Morrison WB, Singleton BA, et al. Medial patellofemoral ligament injury following acute transient dislocation of the patella: MR findings with surgical correlation in 14 patients. J Comput Assist Tomogr 2001;25(6):957–62.
36. Mettler FA Jr, Huda W, Yoshizumi TT, et al. Effective doses in radiology and diagnostic nuclear medicine: a catalog. Radiology 2008;248(1):254–63.
37. Seyahi A, Atalar AC, Koyuncu LO, et al. [Blumensaat line and patellar height]. Acta Orthop Traumatol Turc 2006;40(3):240–7.
38. Wagenaar FC, Koeter S, Anderson PG, et al. Conventional radiography cannot replace CT scanning in detecting tibial tubercle lateralisation. Knee 2007; 14(1):51–4.
39. Tanaka MJ, Elias JJ, Williams AA, et al. Correlation between changes in tibial tuberosity—trochlear groove distance and patellar position during active knee extension on dynamic kinematic computed tomography imaging. Arthroscopy 2015;31(9):1748–55.
40. Brady JM, Rosencrans AS, Shubin Stein BE. Use of TT-PCL versus TT-TG. Curr Rev Musculoskelet Med 2018;11(2):261–5.
41. Camp CL, Stuart MJ, Krych AJ, et al. CT and MRI measurements of tibial tubercle-trochlear groove distances are not equivalent in patients with patellar instability. Am J Sports Med 2013;41(8):1835–40.
42. Seitlinger G, Scheurecker G, Hogler R, et al. Tibial tubercle-posterior cruciate ligament distance: a new measurement to define the position of the tibial tubercle in patients with patellar dislocation. Am J Sports Med 2012;40(5):1119–25.
43. Diederichs G, Issever AS, Scheffler S. MR imaging of patellar instability: injury patterns and assessment of risk factors. Radiographics 2010;30(4):961–81.
44. Cosgarea AJ. Measuring coronal (mal)alignment for patients with patellar instability: tibial tubercle-to-trochlear groove versus tibial tubercle-to-posterior cruciate ligament distance. Arthroscopy 2017;33(11):2035–7.
45. Biedert RM, Albrecht S. The patellotrochlear index: a new index for assessing patellar height. Knee Surg Sports Traumatol Arthrosc 2006;14(8):707–12.
46. Tanaka MJ, Elias JJ, Williams AA, et al. Characterization of patellar maltracking using dynamic kinematic CT imaging in patients with patellar instability. Knee Surg Sports Traumatol Arthrosc 2016;24(11):3634–41.

Coronal Malalignment—
When and How to Perform a
Tibial Tubercle Osteotomy

Elizabeth C. Gardner, MD*, David A. Molho, MD,
John P. Fulkerson, MD

KEYWORDS

- Patellar instability • Tibial tubercle osteotomy • Anteromedialization
- Distal realignment • Anterior knee pain • Patella maltracking • Anteromedial TTO
- Distalization

KEY POINTS

- Distal tibial tubercle realignment osteotomy is often necessary with or without soft tissue procedures for optimal treatment of patella instability and/or pain.
- Medial or anteromedialization tibial tubercle osteotomy (TTO) is effective for adjustment of patella maltracking.
- Anteromedial TTO unloads the patella while adjusting patella alignment in a multiplanar fashion.
- Distalization may be used to address patella alta either in isolation or in combination with medial or anteromedial TTO.
- Anteriorization TTO unloads the patella, particularly the distal pole, without realigning.

INTRODUCTION

Tibial tubercle osteotomies (TTOs) are well-described techniques to treat a range of patellofemoral disorders, including patellofemoral instability, as well as cartilage injury ranging from focal chondral lesions of the patella and trochlea to patellofemoral arthritis. The goal of the procedure is to either alter tracking of the patellofemoral joint or unload its cartilage; in many cases, both may be appropriate. With improved understanding of the complex interplay of its osseous anatomy, the soft tissue structures, and dynamic muscle stability, distal realignment procedures have evolved to be a critical tool in the treatment of common patellofemoral disorders.

Department of Orthopaedic Surgery and Rehabilitation, Yale University, Yale University School of Medicine, 47 College Street, New Haven, CT 06510, USA
* Corresponding author.
E-mail address: elizabeth.gardner@yale.edu
Twitter: @TotalHipKnee (D.A.M.); @patelladoc (J.P.F.)

Clin Sports Med 41 (2022) 15–26
https://doi.org/10.1016/j.csm.2021.07.008
0278-5919/22/Published by Elsevier Inc.

Roux[1] reported the first distal realignment in 1888. Describing a medial transfer of the lateral half of the patella tendon, in addition to medial retinacular plication and lateral release, it was intended to treat patella instability. Goldthwait[2] described a similar procedure nearly concurrently, and thus this medialization became known as the Roux-Goldthwait procedure.

With time, further modifications to Roux' original technique have been described. In order to reduce contact pressures and treat lateral overload, Trillat and colleagues[3] described the technique first used by Elmslie, which involved a flat axial plane osteotomy of the tibial tubercle for medial transfer—this osteotomy has become known as the Elmslie-Trillat procedure.

In 1938, Hauser[4] proposed a modification of the Roux-Goldthwait procedure, including a distal and medial shift of the patella to further increase constraint and reduce the risk of lateral instability. Unfortunately, despite good short-term effects on stability, this resulted in deleterious effects on cartilage contact pressures and resulted in patellofemoral arthritis.[5] Therefore, this procedure has become essentially obsolete, but it still serves as an important reminder of the potential long-term sequelae of distal realignment procedures. Specifically, it underscores the importance of avoiding joint overconstraint in order to prevent future degenerative joint disease.

For pain associated with patellofemoral arthritis, in 1981 Maquet[6] first described a straight anteriorization osteotomy, with the goal of decreasing the cartilage contact pressure. It was ultimately Fulkerson[7] in 1983 who popularized the idea of an antero-medialization, both elevating and medializing the tibial tubercle in a titratable multiplanar osteotomy. Biomechanical models have shown that anteromedialization decreases chondral contact pressure on the lateral patellar facet, which may allow pain relief in some patients with concurrent patellar instability.[8]

Multiplanar osteotomies allow the orthopedic surgeon to individually tailor the procedure to most appropriately address the specific pathoanatomy of the patient. Important considerations include clinical instability history, increased tibial tubercle-trochlear groove (TT-TG) distance, patella alta/baja, and chondral injury. However, this makes it essential that the surgeon has a complete understanding of the complex biomechanical workings of the patellofemoral joint, in order to indicate and treat these patients (**Fig. 1**).

INDICATIONS

The indications for TTO determine the specific procedure design. Although treatment of an acute, first-time lateral patella dislocation continues to evolve, the current standard-of-care treatment remains nonoperative; the most common exception to this is the presence of an unstable osteochondral lesion. TTO is rarely indicated for first-time patella dislocators. Appropriate conservative treatment includes bracing, nonsteroidal antiinflammatory drugs, physical therapy, injection, and patella taping. Physical therapy should focus on closed chain exercises, core and vastus medialis strengthening, balance, and proprioceptive training. The overall reported rate of recurrence after nonoperative management of a first-time traumatic patella dislocation is 33%.[9] Risk factors for recurrent instability include younger age at the time of index dislocation, open physes, sports-related injuries, patella alta, and trochlear dysplasia.[10] In their study, Lewallen and colleagues[10] reported that in those younger than 25 years of age with trochlear dysplasia, the recurrence rate was as high as 69%. In predictive modeling of risk of recurrent dislocation after a first-time event in children and adolescents, Jaquith and colleagues[11] found that the presence of all 4 of their risk factors—a history of contralateral patellar dislocation, patella alta, trochlear dysplasia,

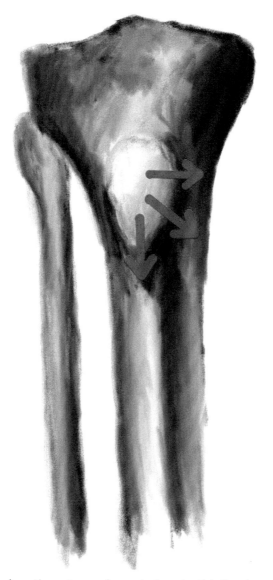

Fig. 1. Tibial tubercle options. Arrows demonstrate potential directions of tibial tubercle translation – distal, medial and anteromedial. (*Courtesy of* David A Molho, MD, New Haven CT.)

and skeletal immaturity—conferred a predicted risk up to 88.4%. Beyond the risk of recurrent instability, the risk of further chondral injury should also be considered. Elias and colleagues[12] reported the frequency of chondral injuries to be as high as 70%. Further considerations in first-time dislocators included the pressures and risks of early return to high-risk sport, as well as more profound malalignment, such that early TTO may be appropriate in certain high-risk patients and clinical scenarios.

Surgical treatment is most commonly indicated for recurrent patella instability or pain despite adequate nonoperative treatment. Surgery will often involve a proximal soft tissue reconstruction procedure in association with a possible distal realignment osteotomy based on patient-specific clinical and radiographic evaluation. In general, a TTO is most commonly considered in patients with an excessive lateral position of the tibial tubercle (most commonly measured by TT-TG >20 mm) or patellar height abnormality (Caton-Deschamps index >1.2). Camp[13] and Tanaka,[14] in separate studies, however, have demonstrated that TT-TG measurements may be variable and potentially inaccurate. Thus, the true utility of TT-TG measurements in isolation is still in question. Rather TT-TG should be considered within the context of the other structural and dynamic factors of the patellofemoral joint, as well as articular damage, in order to identify those patients for which realignment at the tubercle level might be appropriate for compensation.

For patellofemoral chondral lesions or osteoarthritis, surgical indications include persistence of pain, swelling, and/or mechanical symptoms despite a course of similar physical therapy and therapeutic modalities. The indications for treatment of iatrogenic medial instability mirror those discussed earlier, with surgery suggested for those with recalcitrant symptoms, and certainly medial transfer of the tibial tubercle would be contraindicated.

In the setting of chondral injury, either acute due to trauma or that related to chronic patellar overload from malalignment, a TTO may or may not be combined with cartilage restoration procedures to aid in unloading the damaged region. In many cases, articular lesions may be unloaded by TTO alone, such that added articular cartilage implantation or chondral autograft or allograft may be avoided.

MEDIALIZATION OF THE TIBIAL TUBERCLE

As in the Roux-Goldthwait procedure, medialization of the tibial tubercle decreases the lateral force vector on the patella. In doing so, the contact pressure on the patella cartilage is shifted, specifically decreasing the force on the lateral facet.[15,16] Therefore, careful inspection of the patellofemoral cartilage surface must be performed, in order to ensure that the resultant force vector will appropriately off-load the area of cartilage injury. Surgical planning for the optimal amount of medialization is most commonly based on the TT-TG distance, but as mentioned earlier, TT-TG is only one factor to consider. Although there is no clear consensus in the literature, postoperative TT-TG goals generally range from 9 to 15 mm.[17–19] Ultimately the amount of medialization may be limited by the amount of bony contact of the transferred tubercle and the intact tibia.

DISTALIZATION OF THE TIBIAL TUBERCLE

Indications for distalization of the tibial tubercle to reduce the risk of recurrent instability include Caton-Deschamps or Insall-Salvati indices greater than 1.2.[20,21] It is important to avoid overdistalization of the tibial tubercle, which can limit knee flexion and increase risk of nonunion or fixation failure The need for isolated distalization is rare, as patella alta is most commonly associated with other osseous pathoanatomy predisposing to instability—therefore, a multiplanar osteotomy is typically indicated. The authors prefer to include distalization as a part of this multiplanar osteotomy when the Caton-Deschamps index is greater than 1.4 mm. The amount of distalization is such that the postoperative Caton-Deschamps index is 1.1 to 1.2 in order to minimize risks of the procedure.

ANTERIORIZATION OF THE TIBIAL TUBERCLE

Anteriorization in isolation is not a stabilizing procedure. Rather, as described by Maquet, it aims to reduce patellofemoral contact pressures and thus decrease pain. This elevation procedure requires autograft or allograft to support the new position of the tubercle. Straight anteriorization is indicated to unload large distal patellar lesions, bipolar kissing chondral lesions, or arthritis in the setting of a normal TT-TG distance (<15 mm). Rue and colleagues[22] reported that anteriorization may be advantageous in patients with medial patella cartilage lesions for which anteromedialization is contraindicated. Anteriorization of 2 cm can reduce the compressive forces across the joint by 50%.[23] However, the risk of pathologic overload of the superior pole of the patella, as well as wound and bone healing complications, must be considered when determining the extent of anteriorization.[24] Based on in vitro studies, the optimal anteriorization is most commonly between 10 and 15 mm.[25,26] Today, anteriorization is most commonly considered as part of a multiplanar anteromedialization osteotomy in order to maximize the benefits of bone to bone healing.

ANTEROMEDIALIZATION OF THE TIBIAL TUBERCLE

The aim of the anteromedialization osteotomy, as originally described by Fulkerson in 1983, is to combine the positive biomechanical effects of the medialization and anteriorization uniplanar osteotomies, while avoiding the shortcomings of each. The long, flat cut of the osteotomy has a large surface area for cancellous bone healing, as well as for providing sufficient room to place 2 to 3 compression screws of adequate size to provide early stability. In addition, the gradual distal taper of the osteotomy reduces risk of a tibia fracture, a potentially devastating complication of any tibial osteotomy. Finally, the variable angle of the osteotomy allows for individualization of the procedure to most appropriately medialize and anteriorize the tibial tubercle, according to patient-specific pathoanatomy. Biomechanical studies have shown that while correcting patella maltracking, anteromedialization also reduces patellofemoral chondral contact pressures.[16]

CONTRAINDICATIONS

The only absolute contraindication to a distal realignment procedure is skeletal immaturity, with a still open proximal tibial physis and tibial tubercle apophysis.[27] Postoperative genu recurvatum has been reported in this population.[28,29] As such, nonsurgical or alternative stabilization procedures, as well as activity modification, should be used until skeletal maturity around the tibial tubercle has been reached.

Relative contraindications vary based on the specific osteotomy proposed. Patients must stop smoking before having a TTO of any sort to minimize risk of delayed or nonunion. A history of medial patellar instability increases the risk of medial subluxation or dislocation following an osteotomy that medializes the tibial tubercle further and thus should be avoided.[30] Because of the shift of contact pressure to the medial facet of the patella with any medialization procedure, patients with focal cartilage lesions of the medial patella or medial trochlea should avoid an isolated medialization osteotomy; transfer in other planes, however, may be performed.[22] Diffuse patellofemoral osteoarthritis portends poor outcomes in patients undergoing distalization procedures.[31–33]

SURGICAL TREATMENT OPTIONS
Anteromedialization of the Tibial Tubercle

Based on clinical examination and imaging, with 3-dimensional imaging and printing whenever possible, one develops a clear concept of where to place the tibial tubercle in order to optimize loads and alignment of the patellofemoral joint. Usual goals are to unload the distal and lateral patella while optimizing stability of the patellofemoral joint. Anteromedialization TTO is most desirable to offload the lateral patella and trochlea for treatment of lateral patellofemoral pain and arthrosis related to overload. It may be indicated together with medial patellofemoral reconstruction for recurrent patella instability related to lateral maltracking and particularly when the distal medial or lateral patella is damaged.

The procedure starts with arthroscopy in the supine position. Standard diagnostic arthroscopy should be performed to assess for concurrent pathology. Specific attention should be made to patellofemoral joint, in both static and dynamic states. It is important to assess the movement of the joint without fluid inflation, as this can affect the position of the patella with respect to the trochlea. At times, patellofemoral tracking may be viewed from the superolateral approach, but in many cases, viewing from a standard anteromedial or anterolateral portal is sufficient to evaluate location and extent of lateral tracking and localize articular lesions. Any necessary chondroplasty may be handled arthroscopically. Visualized lateral patella tilt, confirmed radiographically, may indicate a need for lateral release or lengthening. Arthroscopic limited lateral release may be needed to permit necessary anterior and medial translation of the patella. In addition, arthroscopic release of infrapatellar contraction within the region of Hoffa fat pad may be necessary before performing bony portions of the procedure.

The anterior skin incision extends from 2 cm above the tibial tuberosity to approximately 6 to 8 cm distal to the tuberosity in most cases but can be shortened or lengthened according to surgeon preference and patient anatomy. Generally, the incision should be positioned just lateral to the tuberosity, such that the final transfer and placement of screws are medial to the incision. The patella tendon insertion is immediately identified deep to the subcutaneous tissues. In order to allow a hemostat to be placed behind the distal patella tendon, incisions are made just medial and lateral to the tendon, just proximal to its insertion onto the tibial tubercle, extending approximately 2 cm proximal to the tuberosity. Another incision is made along the tibialis anterior attachment to the proximal-lateral tibia, and a Cobb elevator is used to elevate the anterior tibialis subperiosteally such that it may be reflected to the posterolateral corner of the tibia. Care should be taken at this time to ensure hemostasis, as well as complete visualization of the entire lateral surface of the tibia in order to protect the surrounding neurovascular structures.

The osteotomy itself must be defined accurately and always tapered distally to the anterior tibial cortex. Guide systems are available from various companies. A Hoffman drill guide may be used also to define the osteotomy plane with multiple drill holes. Some surgeons may do the osteotomy free hand but this normally requires a lot of experience because of the multiple planes affected by the single cut. No matter which technique is used, paramount to safely performing a TTO is close observation of drill tips or saw cut as they come through the lateral tibial cortex, with protection of the neurovascular structures behind a retractor. It is often best to start any drilling or cutting distally where the osteotomy is most anterior and easily viewed.

After initial planning of the osteotomy, the surgeon must confirm that biomechanical result will be as desired, dialing in more or less anteriorization and medialization based on the angle of the osteotomy plane. Once the planned cut is optimized, the osteotomy cut begins distally, always assuring the osteotomy will exit the anterolateral tibia at the tibial crest in to avoid a step-off or stress riser. The steeper the osteotomy, the further posterior the exit plane will be on the lateral tibia. So this cut must be watched closely, always in full view and never allowed to go posterior toward the anterior tibial artery and the deep peroneal nerve. Most osteotomies are designed at about a 45° angle to the transverse plane of the tibia. Steeper cuts will allow more anteriorization and less medialization. The surgeon should always be thinking of the location and extent of patella and trochlea articular lesions as well as the patellofemoral tracking pattern, designing the angle to optimize unloading and aligning benefits of anteromedialization. The osteotomy cut must taper anteriorly at its distal extent. It should extend proximally through the medial cortex to approximately 5 mm above the patella tendon insertion proximomedially. The proximal extent of the osteotomy laterally is determined largely by the angle of the cut. In a steep osteotomy, the lateral exit for the osteotomy may be well behind the patella tendon. The lateral exit for the osteotomy should always be under direct vision and anterior to the posterolateral corner of the tibia.

Next, a large straight osteotomy is used proximally to connect the earlier cuts made with a saw. First, the posterolateral osteotomy cut is connected with the proximal cut made 5 mm above the lateral patellar tendon insertion. Then another cut is made proximal to the patella tendon insertion, connecting the medial and lateral osteotomy cuts, thus freeing the osteotomy fragment. A green stick fracture of its distal tip of the osteotomy permits an anterior and medial rotation of the fragment. If the osteotomy has been done properly, the fragment will rotate anteromedially on a perfectly flat plane. In most cases, the bone will rotate approximately 1 cm, as measured at its proximal extent. At this point, with provisional fixation in place, it is imperative to assess the unloading effect and the resultant alignment within the joint. The arthroscope should be reintroduced into the joint to assess both the static and dynamic effects. Again, it is important that this is assessed in a dry joint. Adjustments to the position of the osteotomy should be made at this time, particularly taking care to avoid overmedialization. After confirming desired unloading and alignment arthroscopically, the osteotomy is secured under compression using 2 fully threaded cortical screws into the posterior tibial cortex, overdrilling, and countersinking the anterior holes slightly to enable a lag effect, as well as to minimize the potential for symptomatic hardware in the future.

Before closure, careful attention should be made to hemostasis. The anterior compartment maybe left open, and the incisions are closed in a layered fashion.

Distalization

When distalization of the tibial tubercle is warranted, the tubercle transfer osteotomy cut may be performed as usual to achieve the desired anteriorization and/or medialization. Before fixation, local metaphyseal cortical bone may be placed above the distalized fragment for buttressing in the desired location.

A preferable modification pushes the tubercle fragment distally as it is transferred anteromedial or medially, and this is accomplished by creating an oblique proximal cut, above the tibial tubercle, designed in a manner to displace the tubercle transfer shingle distally as it is moved anteromedially or medially. It is possible to achieve 5 to 10 mm of distalization quite easily with this modification, and the resulting construct is very secure without the need to add bone graft. Resection of a small amount of the distal tip of the osteotomy fragment is performed to avoid subcutaneous prominence. With this technique, a proximal buttress is achieved making the distalization quite stable (**Fig. 2**).

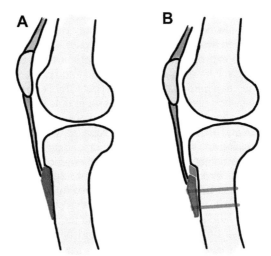

Fig. 2. Distalization of the patella. (A) Pre-surgical state. (B) Post-surgical state, with a proximal buttress to the distalized fragment. (*Courtesy of* David A Molho, MD, New Haven CT.)

Following distalization, the rehabilitation program must be altered because of increased pressure in flexion.[34] Consequently the time to full flexion is delayed 2 to 3 weeks to avoid avulsion of the tubercle transfer shingle.

Straight Medialization

Sometimes called the Elmslie-Trillat procedure, straight medial transfer of the tibial tubercle requires a transverse cut deep to the tibial tubercle. The osteotomy is otherwise the same as performed for an anteromedial tibial tubercle transfer but risks adding load to a medial or distal patella articular lesion. Both of these lesions are common after patella dislocation, particularly in the presence of preexisting lateral maltracking of the patella. Straight medialization of the tibial tubercle generally creates a smaller shingle of bone in most cases and thus is particularly desirable for a more severe lateral tracking extensor mechanism, in which more than 1 cm of medialization is necessary to achieve lasting stability.

Anteriorization of the Tibial Tubercle

Although isolated anteriorization of the tibial tubercle is uncommon, it may be accomplished via several techniques. The first is the original Maquet procedure. However, this requires excessive distraction of the osteotomized fragment and is generally contraindicated; therefore, it will not be further described here.

The authors recommend that anteriorization be performed using a modification of the standard anteromedialization technique, which is familiar and comfortable to most surgeons. After performing the oblique osteotomy as described earlier, a piece of local metaphyseal cortical bone graft is placed posterior to the elevated osteotomized fragment after moving it about 8 mm along the osteotomy plane. The effect of this is to offset the osteotomy fragment laterally, thus neutralizing the effect of the osteotomy cut and resulting in a straight anteriorization effect (**Fig. 3**).

Some surgeons have advocated for a sagittal plane osteotomy, with bone graft placed beneath it for anteriorization. Common criticism of this technique is the very

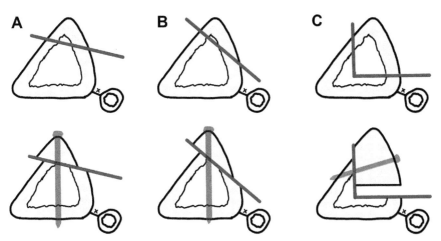

Fig. 3. Cross-sections of osteotomy cuts. (A) Shallow oblique osteotomy of anteromedialization. (B) Steep oblique osteotomy of anteromedialization with resulting more anteriorization. (C) Offset osteotomy to neutralize medialization and result in pure anteriorization. (*Courtesy of* David A Molho, MD, New Haven CT.)

large size of the osteotomy fragment, which can weaken the proximal tibia excessively.

For all anteriorization procedures, one must be careful not to elevate the fragment excessively, in order to avoid pressure on the skin and the danger of wound dehiscence.

POSTOPERATIVE MANAGEMENT

Postoperatively patients should use crutches for at least 6 to 8 weeks after surgery, starting with limited weight-bearing and progressing toward full weight-bearing at about 6 weeks postoperation. This protection is necessary to prevent a proximal tibial fracture, the occurrence of which is relatively high with early weight-bearing protocols.[35] While ambulating in the early post-operative phase, the knee should be kept in full extension in either a knee immobilizer or a hinged knee brace locked in extension. However, early seated range of motion, starting as early as postoperative day 1, is recommended to prevent arthrofibrosis. The patient should do at least one cycle of motion each day with a goal of 90° flexion at 4 weeks and full motion by 8 weeks.

COMPLICATIONS

Servien and colleagues[18] reported the overall complication rate following distal realignment procedures to be 7.4%. In a review by Payne and colleagues,[36] in which the relatively morbid Maquet procedure was excluded, the other methods of tibial tubercle transfer procedures had a combined complication rate of 4.6%. The most reported "complication" is symptomatic hardware, with as many as 50% of patients undergoing removal of hardware for this.[37,38] However, hardware removal sometimes is planned at the preference of the patient and surgeon, so it might not be considered a complication. Minor complications, such as delayed wound healing, superficial wound infection, and skin irritation, have been reported and are generally treated nonsurgically.[39] The use of compression screw fixation limits the risk of nonunion at the osteotomy site to 3.7%.[40,41] Nonunions are likely related to smoking, imperfect osteotomy, insufficient fixation, or lack of patient compliance in the authors' experience. However, because the osteotomy site is a stress riser, a period of protected weight-bearing is still essential to prevent a proximal tibia fracture.[42–44] Although fortunately rare, compartment syndrome has been reported, and surgeons must work to ensure adequate hemostasis and remain vigilant for this potentially disastrous complication.[45] Leaving the anterior compartment open after the osteotomy virtually eliminates this risk. Venous thromboembolic events, including both pulmonary embolism[46] and deep venous thromboembolism,[43] have also been reported; however, the role of standard chemoprophylaxis is not clear. Other less common postoperative complications include medial patellar dislocation, arthrofibrosis, symptomatic neuroma, anterior tibial artery or deep peroneal nerve injury, or osteomyelitis.[20,21] Nonetheless, Klinge[47] reported sustained good results of anteromedialization TTO at a minimum of 15-year follow-up.

SUMMARY

Distal tibial tubercle realignment procedures provide versatile options for the orthopedic surgeon treating patellofemoral instability, associated chondral injuries, and lateral patellofemoral arthrosis. TTOs for cases of lateral patella instability are often combined with proximal soft tissue patella stabilization procedures and cartilage restoration. It is incumbent on the surgeon to accurately assess the patient's entire pathoanatomy in order to most appropriately determine the direction and obliquity of the osteotomy and transfer to optimize the outcome in both the short- and long-term.

ACKNOWLEDGMENTS

The authors would like to thank Dr David Molho for the use of his illustrations in this article.

DISCLOSURE

The authors have nothing to disclose.

REFERENCES

1. Roux C. Recurrent dislocation of the patella: operative treatment. 1888. Clin Orthop Relat Res 2006;452:17–20.
2. Goldthwait JE. Permanent dislocation of the patella. The report of a case of twenty years' duration, successfully treated by transplantation of the patella tendons with the tubercle of the tibia. Ann Surg 1899;29(1):62–8.
3. Trillat A, Dejour H, Couette A. Diagnosis and treatment of recurrent dislocations of the patella. Rev Chir Orthop Reparatrice Appar Mot 1964;50:813–24.
4. Hauser E. Total tendon transplantation for slipping patella. Surg Gynecol Obstet 1938;66:199–214.
5. Christman OD, Snook GA, Wilson TC. A long-term prospective study of the Hauser and Roux-Goldthwaite procedures for recurrent patellar dislocation. Clin Orthop Relat Res 1979;144:27–30.
6. Radin EL. The Macquet procedure – anterior displacement of the tibial tubercle. Indications, contraindication, and precautions. Clin Orthop Relat Res 1986;213:241–8.
7. Fulkerson JP. Anteromedialization of the tibial tuberosity for patellofemoral malalignment. Clin Orthop Relat Res 1983;177:176–81.

8. Saranathan A, Kirkpatrick MS, Mani S, et al. The effect of tibial tuberosity realignment procedures on the patellofemoral pressure distrubtion. Knee Surg Sports Tramatol Arthrosc 2021;20(10):2054–61.

9. Erickson BJ, Mascareenhas R, Sayegh ET, et al. Does operative treatment of first-time patellar dislocations lead to increased patellofemoral stability? A systemic review of overlapping meta-analyses. Arthroscopy 2015;31:1207–15.

10. Lewallen L, McIntosh A, Dahm D. First-time patellofemoral dislocation: risk factors for recurrent instability. J Knee Surg 2015;28:303–10.

11. Jaquith BP, Parikh SN. Predictors of recurrent patellar instability in children and adolescents after first-time dislocation. J Pediatr Orthop 2017;37:484–90.

12. Elias DA, White LM, Fithian DC. Acute lateral patellar dislocation at MR imaging: injury patterns of medial patellar soft-tissue restraints and osteochondral injuries of the inferomedial patella. Radiology 2002;225:736–43.

13. Camp CL, Stuart MJ, Krych AJ, et al. CT and MRI measurements of tibial tubercle-trochlear groove distances are not equivalent in patients with patellar instability. Am J Sports Med 2013;41(8):1835–40.

14. Tanaka MJ, Cosgarae AJ. Measuring malalignment on imaging in the treatment of patellofemoral instability. Am J Orthop 2017;46(3):148–51.

15. Kuroda R, Kambic H, Vealdevit A, et al. Articular cartilage contact pressure after tibial tubercle transfer: a cadaveric study. Am J Sports Med 2001;29(4):7.

16. Ramappa AJ, Apreleva M, Harrold FR, et al. The effects of medialization and anteromedialization of the tibial tubercle on patellofemoral mechanics and kinematics. Am J Sports Med 2006;34(5):749–56.

17. Dejour D, Le Coultre B. Osteotomies in patella-femoral instabilities. Sports Med Arthrosc Rev 2007;15:8.

18. Servien E, Verdonk PC, Neyret P. Tibial tuberosity transfer for episodic patellar dislocation. Sports Med Arthrosc Rev 2007;15(2):7.

19. Tecklenburg K, Feller JA, Whitehead TS, et al. Outcome of surgery for recurrent patellar dislocation based on the distance of the tibial tuberosity to the trochlea groove. J Bone Joint Surg Br 2010;92:5.

20. Cootjans K, Dujardin J, Vandenneucker H, et al. A surgical algorithm for the treatment of recurrent patellar dislocation: results at 5 year follow-up. Acta Orthop Belg 2013;79:318–25.

21. Feller JA. Distal realignment (tibial tubercle transfer). Sports Med Arthrosc Rev 2012;20:10.

22. Rue JP, Colton A, Zare SM, et al. Trochlear contact pressures after straight anteriorization of the tibial tuberosity. Am J Sports Med 2008;36(10):7.

23. Maquet P. A biomechanical treatment of femoro-patellar arthrosis: Advancement of the patellar tendon. Rev Rhum Al Osteoartic 1963;30:779–83.

24. Maquet P. Advancement of the tibial tuberosity. Clin Orthop Relat Res 1976;115:225–30.

25. Fernandez L, Usabiaga J, Yubero J, et al. An experimental study of the redistribution of patellofemoral pressures by the anterior displacement of the anterior tuberosity of the tibia. Clin Orthop Relat Res 1989;238:183–9.

26. Akgun U, Nuran R, Karahan M. Modified Fulkerson osteotomy in recurrent patellofemoral dislocations. Acta Orthop Traumatol Turc 2010;44:27–35.

27. Hinton RY, Sharma KM. Acute and recurrent patellar instability in the young athlete. Orthop Clin North Am 2003;34(3):385–96.

28. Harrison MH. The results of a realignment operation for recurrent dislocation of the patella. J Bone Joint Surg Br 1955;37(4):559–67.

29. Macnab I. Recurrent dislocation of the patella. J Bone Joint Surg Am 1952; 34(4):11.
30. Bicos J, Fulkerson JP. Indications and technique of distal tubercle anteromedialization. Operat Tech Orthop 2007;17(4):223–33.
31. Piroriano AJ, Weinstein RN, Buck DA, et al. Correlation of patellar articular lesions with results from anteromedial tibial tubercle transfer. Am J Sports Med 1997; 25(4):5.
32. Pritsch T, Haim A, Arbel R, et al. Tailored tibial tubercle transfer for patellofemoral malalignment; analysis of clinical outcomes. Knee Surg Sports Traumatol Arthrosc 2007;15(8):994–1002.
33. Wang CJ, Chan YS, Chen HH, et al. Factors affecting the outcome of distal realignment for patellofemoral disorders of the knee. Knee 2005;12(3):195–200.
34. Koh J, Jones T, Elias JJ. Tibial tubercle distalization reduces contact pressures in patella alta and instability. Arthroscopy 2021;37(1, Supp):E82–3.
35. Smith TO, Song F, Donell ST, et al. Operative versus non-operative management of patellar dislocation. A meta-analysis. Knee Surg Sports Traumatol Arthrosc 2011;19(6):988–98.
36. Payne J, Rimmke N, Schmitt LC, et al. The incidence of complications of tibial tubercle osteotomy: a systematic review. Arthroscopy 2015;31(9):1819–25.
37. Koeter S, Diks MJ, Anderson PG, et al. A modified tibial tubercle osteotomy for patellar maltracking: results at two years. J Bone Joint Surg Br 2002;84:4.
38. Tjoumakaris FP, Forsythe B, Bradley JP. Patellofemoral instability in athletes: treatment via modified Fulkerson osteotomy and lateral release. Am J Sports Med 2010;38(5):992–9.
39. Middleton KK, Gruber S, Shubin Stein BE. Why and where to move the tibial tubercle: indications and techniques for tibial tubercle osteotomy. Sports Med Arthrosc Rev 2019;27(4):154–60.
40. Farr J, Schepsis A, Cole B, et al. Anteromedialization: review and technique. J Knee Surg 2007;20(2):120–8.
41. Mayer C, Magnusesen RA, Servien E, et al. Patellar tendon tenodesis in association with tibial tubercle distalization for the treatment of episodic patellar dislocation with patella alta. Am J Sports Med 2012;40(2):345–51.
42. Farr J. Tibial tubercle osteotomy. Tech Knee Surg 2003;2(1):28–42.
43. Fulkerson JP, Becker GJ, Meaney JA, et al. Anteromedial tibial tubercle transfer without bone graft. Am J Sports Med 1990;18(5):490–6 [discussion: 496–7].
44. Bellemans J, Cauwenberghs F, Brys P, et al. Fracture of the proximal tibia after Fulkerson anteromedial tibia tubercle transfer: a report of four cases. Am J Sports Med 1998;26(2):300–2.
45. Cox JS. Evaluation of the Roux-Elmslie-Trillat procedure for knee extensor realignment. Am J Sports Med 1982;10(5):303–10.
46. Wiggins HE. The anterior tibial compartment syndrome: a complication of the Hauser procedure. Clin Orthop Relat Res 1975;113:90–4.
47. Klinge S, Fulkerson J. Fifteen year follow-up of anteromedial tibial tubercle transfer for lateral patellofemoral arthritis. Arthroscopy 2019;35(7):2146–51.

Rotational Deformity— When and How to Address Femoral Anteversion and Tibial Torsion

Benjamin Noonan, MD[a], Trenton Cooper, DO[b],
Michael Chau, MD[c], Melissa Albersheim, MD[c],
Elizabeth A. Arendt, MD[c], Marc Tompkins, MD[c],*

KEYWORDS

- Patellofemoral instability • Femoral version • Tibial torsion • Derotation osteotomy

KEY POINTS

- Axial plane malalignment is an important factor to consider in patients with patellofemoral instability.
- Surgeons should be familiar with the examination and work up to evaluate rotational deformities.
- There are many locations and methods to surgically address rotational malalignment and surgeons should have an understanding of the various options to best address an individual patient.

INTRODUCTION

The patellofemoral (PF) joint is composed of the posterior surface of the patella as well as the trochlear surface of the distal anterior femur. The complexity of this joint—with multiple bony contact points as well as sites of soft tissue attachment—predisposes it to numerous mechanisms for instability. Patellar instability may be seen in a wide age range with various etiologies including an acute traumatic event, generalized ligament laxity, patella alta, or trochlear dysplasia.[1] Patellar instability, including patellar subluxations and lateral patellar dislocations, may also be the result of rotational abnormalities of both the femur and the tibia, including excessive femoral anteversion and external tibial torsion.

---

[a] Sanford Orthopedics & Sports Medicine, 2301 25th Street South, Fargo, ND 58103, USA;
[b] Gillette Children's Specialty Healthcare, 200 University Avenue East, St Paul, MN 55101, USA;
[c] Department of Orthopedic Surgery, University of Minnesota, 2450 Riverside Avenue South, Suite R 200, Minneapolis, MN 55454, USA
* Corresponding author.
E-mail address: marc.tompkins@tria.com

Clin Sports Med 41 (2022) 27–46
https://doi.org/10.1016/j.csm.2021.07.011
0278-5919/22/© 2021 Elsevier Inc. All rights reserved.

Lower extremity torsion has been documented in the literature starting back in 1903 by Pierre Germain Marie Le Damany with his description of limb torsion.[2] Today, tibial rotation is most commonly recognized as the relationship between the transcondylar and transmalleolar axes.[3–6] During fetal development, the tibia is internally rotated due to limb bud development and intrauterine positioning.[7] At birth, the tibia undergoes external rotation gradually until skeletal maturity is reached, with most rotation occurring during the first 4 years of development.[8] Femoral anteversion is defined as the axis of the femoral neck and femoral condyles in the transverse plane.[9] The established average femoral anteversion at birth is 40°, which decreases during development until approximately age 8 years.[10] Although the definitions of femoral anteversion and tibial torsion are well accepted, what is considered within the range of normal limits is more controversial with a wide variation of reported normal anatomy and accepted measurement values. For average adult tibial rotation, the literature ranges from 0° to 47°.[8,11] The average femoral anteversion documented in the literature varies by up to 30°.[9]

Currently, there is no standardization of what degree of deviation from "normal" meets criteria for surgical intervention. Although derotational osteotomies are established treatment methods to correct osseous axial plane malalignments, the surgical indications are unclear because of the previously stated diversity of definitions for "normal" axial plane rotation. Surgical decision-making becomes more complex with the diversity of techniques and anatomic axes for measuring femoral and tibial torsion. This article seeks to provide an overview of the current knowledge and approaches to dealing with this challenging topic.

BIOMECHANICS
Femur

Abnormal transverse plane alignment can lead to many alterations in the typical function of the lower limb and can have tremendous effects on the PF joint. This can result in magnified contact forces, altered kinematics of the PF joint, and dynamics in the lower limb, which can lead to not only PF dysfunction/pain, but also instability.[12] To improve the coverage of the femoral head by the acetabulum, many patients with femoral anteversion will have a compensatory dynamic internal rotation of the hip. This results in transverse plane changes of the entire femoral segment, including the knee, and alterations in PF function.[13–15] Biomechanical cadaveric studies have demonstrated that when compared with the unrotated state, internal rotation of the femur leads to a lateral center of force shift along with increased patellar tilt.[13] As the trochlea is medialized, there is a relative lateral translation of the patella compared to the medialized trochlea.[12,13] Compensatory internal hip rotation also causes dynamic knee valgus and proximal (hip) weakness.[16] Patellofemoral mechanics are disrupted including a varus moment at the knee with a resultant lateral vector on the patella.[17] A laterally directed force vector on the patella leads to increased contact forces on the lateral PF joint and elevated risk for lateral instability.

Tibia

Abnormal torsional alignment of the tibia, specifically external tibial torsion, has also been associated with abnormal PF mechanics and instability. Typically, external tibial torsion leads to an external foot progression angle. The foot being out of plane with the line of progression leads to changes in the typical axis of the knee. This results in abnormal knee forces, primarily a varus moment, or valgus position.[18] Turner measured tibial torsion in greater than 800 consecutive patients and found patients with patellar instability had a significantly increased external tibial torsion; this was felt likely to be due to changes in the ground reaction forces leading to deviations in the direction of external loading of the limb.[19] Schwartz and Lakin demonstrated that external tibial torsion leads to flexion, valgus, and external rotation accelerations of the knee joint. This leads to lever arm dysfunction and decreases the ability of the soleus to extend the knee.[20] These dynamic changes in gait can alter the kinematics and kinetics of the PF joint and place the patella in an environment that can result in patellar instability.

HISTORY

Identifying torsional abnormalities is classically discovered on physical examination and/or radiographs, but there may be a few aspects of the history that may provide suspicion of a transverse plane abnormality. A history of "W" sitting may be described during childhood and may suggest persistent femoral anteversion. Inquiring about foot progression can also assist in the identification of a potential torsional issue:

- In-toeing
  - Femoral anteversion
  - Internal tibial torsion
- Out-toeing
  - External tibial torsion

A full medical history should be obtained as well as inquiring about genetic or neuromuscular diagnoses. For example, patients with cerebral palsy, myelomeningocele, and Down syndrome have a higher likelihood of transverse plane abnormalities.

PHYSICAL EXAMINATION

Paramount to the identification of lower extremity torsional pathology is a thorough physical examination. Although the history may provide some insight, typically the first identification of a possible torsional issue derives from the examination and can identify the need for further workup (radiographs/gait analysis). The examination should include:

- Gait:
  - Foot progression angle
    - In-toeing: femoral anteversion
    - Out-toeing: external tibial torsion
  - Internal rotation of the hip in stance and medial pointing "squinting" patella
- Standing with both patellae forward:
  - Coronal plane alignment (genu varum/valgum)
  - Position of feet in or out may be an indication of tibial torsion
- Prone examination:
  - Internal > external hip rotation suggests femoral anteversion
  - Trochanteric prominence angle (**Fig. 1**)
    - There are limitations in terms of reproducibility; although quite good consistency has been noted with intraobserver examination measurements, interobserver examination measurements have shown less consistency.[10,21–25]
  - Thigh foot angle (**Fig. 2**), bimalleolar axis, second toe test.[25–27]
    - Foot must be held in a subtalar neutral position
- Foot examination:
  - Pes planus

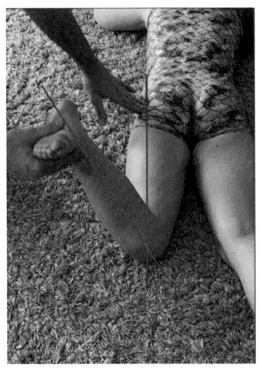

Fig. 1. The trochanteric prominence angle is measured with the greater trochanter palpated laterally in the midsagittal plane. The angle formed by a vertical line and the tibia results in the trochanteric prominence angle.

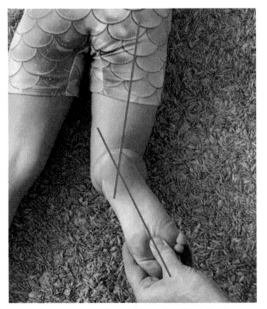

Fig. 2. The thigh foot angle is measured with the subtalar joint in neutral and the knee at 90°. It is measured as the angle between the foot and thigh.

- In isolation, typically leads to an external foot progression angle and may lead to a false diagnosis of external tibial torsion
- Femoral anteversion: Pes planus may mask the typical in-toeing and may have a normal foot progression angle
  o Hyperlaxity (Beighton Scale)
    - Although not directly related to the bony pathology, it is important to understand if hyperlaxity is contributing to axial plane malalignment because excess rotation can occur through the knee joint.

IMAGING AND DIAGNOSTIC WORKUP

Technological measurements of femoral version and tibial torsion are determined by user-defined reference axes at the proximal and distal ends of each bone. These reference axes are conventionally based on historically described anthropometric parameters in cadaveric specimens.[28] For the femur, the femoral neck axis is defined as the line between the center of the head and base of the neck, and the bicondylar axis is defined as the line tangential to the posterior aspects of the femoral condyles.[29,30] For the tibia, the transcondylar axis is defined by the line that passes through the centers of the medial and lateral joint surfaces, and the bimalleolar axis is defined as the line between the midpoints of the ankle malleoli.[2,5] Measurement validity and reliability can be influenced by discrepancies in defining these reference axes.

Computed Tomography

Computed tomography (CT) is the current gold standard for measuring lower extremity rotation because of its ability to distinctly visualize osseous landmarks in the axial plane. Various techniques for defining reference axes have been described to measure femoral anteversion and tibial torsion.[3,31] Although intraobserver and interobserver reliabilities have been robust for most techniques, the actual measurements of rotation can differ substantially depending on the selected reference axes, especially at the proximal femur and proximal tibia.[32–34] For femoral anteversion, the single-slice CT method just distal to the femoral head has been shown to be the most accurate, although this remains controversial.[31,34] (**Fig. 3**). For tibial torsion, CT cuts within 2 cm of the proximal tibial articular surface have been shown to be

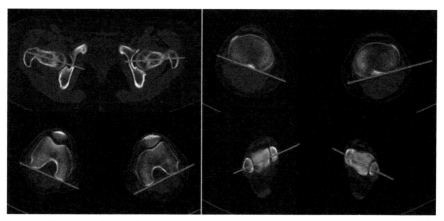

Fig. 3. In this example, the femoral version is measured between the femoral neck and the posterior condylar axis. The tibial torsion is measured between the posterior condylar and bimalleolar axes.

reliable regardless of the selected reference axis (posterior condylar, transcondylar, or anterior condylar)[3] (see **Fig. 3**). It is essential to keep in mind that difficulty with patient positioning, for example, because of joint contractures, nonspherical femoral head deformity, valgus neck-shaft angle, short neck, and greater torsional severity can cause inaccurate and imprecise CT measurements in the axial plane, potentially resulting in misdiagnoses or surgical planning errors.[34]

Magnetic Resonance Imaging

Magnetic resonance imaging (MRI) is an alternative to CT for measuring lower extremity rotation that spares patients of ionizing radiation and additionally provides high-resolution imaging of soft tissue structures.[35] The measurement techniques are similar for both modalities and have been shown to have a strong correlation.[10,36–39] It should be noted, however, that multiple authors have reported femoral anteversion determined by CT to be consistently higher than femoral anteversion determined by MRI, and these values can reach clinical significance.[10,37,39] The disadvantages of MRI include high cost, incompatibility with certain metal implants, and longer acquisition time, which may lead to motion artifacts and require patients to be sedated during the procedure.

Low-Dose Biplanar Radiography (EOS Imaging)

EOS imaging enables axial plane analysis of the lower extremity by 3-dimensional reconstruction of biplanar radiographs, parametric modeling, and statistical inferencing using the SterEOS software[40] (**Fig. 4**). Patients must be able to stand upright in a

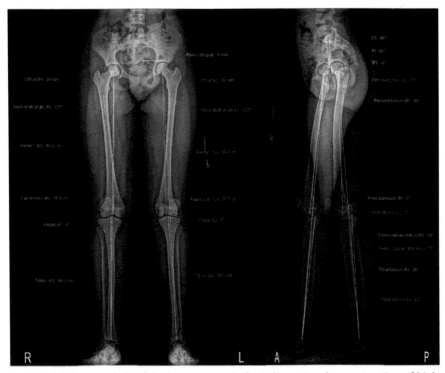

Fig. 4. Axial plane analysis of the lower extremity by 3-dimensional reconstruction of biplanar radiographs, parametric modeling, and statistical inferencing via EOS imaging.

slot scanner. Digital radiographs in both coronal and sagittal planes are simultaneously acquired from the pelvis to feet with the legs in a staggered stance to avoid overlap in the lateral view. The 3-dimensional reconstruction process is a software-guided step-by-step protocol that generates osseous envelopes by identifying the femoral head and neck, greater and lesser trochanters, femoral condyles, tibial plateaus, and ankle malleoli. Axial plane parameters are automatically calculated by the software, including femoral anteversion, femorotibial rotation, and tibial torsion. The accuracy and precision of EOS imaging in measuring femoral anteversion and tibial torsion have been demonstrated to be comparable to CT and MRI.[41–47] The main advantage of EOS imaging is its ability to provide a comprehensive evaluation of lower extremity alignment with substantially lower ionizing radiation exposure compared with conventional radiography (3–43 times) and CT (4–87 times), where absorbed doses vary depending on anatomic site and organ as well as the selected EOS protocol.[28] These advantages also favor its potential to be used for postoperative evaluation with a low cost, low radiation option. Potential limitations of EOS imaging include patient positioning error, for example, inadvertently superimposing anatomic landmarks on the lateral projection, postprocessing user error, motion artifacts, high capital expense, difficulty in obtaining 3-dimensional models of patients with severe deformities or who cannot stand still during the scan, and a manufacturer caution that children younger than 15 years may lack the fully developed osseous landmarks needed for accurate measurements.[48–50]

Gait Analysis

Gait analysis is the quantitative measurement of human kinematics, or geometry of joint motion, that is typically used for evaluating gait disorders.[26] (**Fig. 5**). The most sophisticated gait analysis methods currently involve optical tracking systems that identify the displacement of markers placed at specific anatomic landmarks. Either 3 active or reflective markers are placed on each lower extremity segment (pelvis, 2 femurs, 2 tibiae, and 2 feet) and a scanner or multiple video cameras are used to capture and plot their relative positions in a computerized 3-dimensional coordinate system.[51] As markers cannot be noninvasively placed inside joints at the center of rotation, which is required to obtain accurate kinematic data, mathematical algorithms have been developed to find the most likely orientation and intersection of all axes by plotting the arc of rotation of each segment followed by interpolating into the center of each arc.[52] Therefore, unlike static imaging modalities, gait analysis not only evaluates structural rotational alignment but also dynamic joint rotation as the body compensates to optimize biomechanical efficiency. When comparing measurements of lower extremity rotation between gait analysis and CT, there is substantially better correlation for tibial torsion than femoral anteversion, which is thought to be predominantly due to compensatory hip rotation.[53]

Radiography

Anteroposterior standing alignment films cannot provide accurate axial plane measurements but does offer a preliminary impression of lower extremity rotation by noting the positions of the lesser trochanters at the hips, intercondylar notch, fibular orientation at the knee, and fibular orientation at the ankle. Fluoroscopic techniques to measure lower extremity rotation are most commonly performed intraoperatively during femoral or tibial shaft fracture fixation. The C-arm machine can be used to measure rotation by orbiting between planes. For the femur, the angle of rotation between true lateral projections of the hip and knee provides a measurement of femoral version.[54] Alternatively, with the posterior femoral condyles flat against the table to

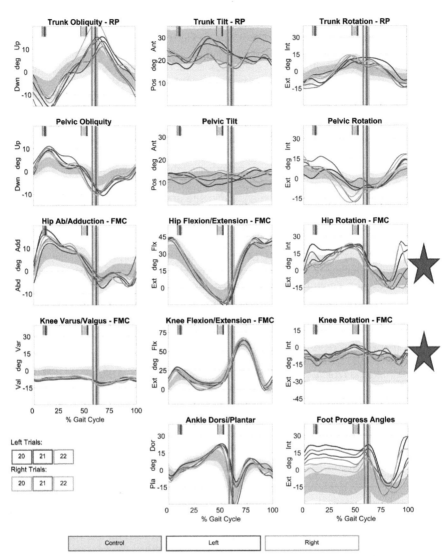

Fig. 5. Gait analysis display, with hip and knee rotation noted by the stars.

set the knee at neutral rotation, the angle of rotation with respect to the table to obtain a perfect lateral projection of the hip provides a measurement of femoral version.[55] For the tibia, the angle of rotation between perfect lateral projections of the knee and ankle provides a measurement of tibial torsion.[56] At present, there is a lack of literature supporting the feasibility of fluoroscopy for measuring lower extremity rotation.

SURGICAL TECHNIQUES
Femoral Osteotomy

Before performing a femoral osteotomy, one must decide on the level of the osteotomy and how much correction to perform. Unfortunately, there is no clear guiding evidence to determine either of these questions.[57] Typical osteotomy locations include proximal, diaphyseal, and distal, each with its own advantages and disadvantages.[57,58] Planned correction is typically based on returning rotational alignment to "normal" values[57] or a balancing of hip internal and external rotation[59] with osteotomies at all levels allowing adequate rotational correction.[60]

Proximal femoral osteotomy

Osteotomies of the proximal femur can be intertrochanteric or subtrochanteric (**Fig. 6**). Benefits of the proximal osteotomy include a single incision and the ability to make large corrections. Potential drawbacks are that it can be more difficult to control coronal plane alignment and restricted weight-bearing may be required depending on the mode of fixation. Proximal intertrochanteric osteotomies have shown durable and favorable clinical outcomes in ambulatory children with cerebral palsy.[61] Hatem and colleagues[62] reported on the outcomes of 37 subtrochanteric osteotomies in 34 patients over a 2-year period. Clinical improvement was demonstrated in 33 hips with 2 hips requiring revision to a larger intramedullary (IM) nail to treat nonunion.

Proximal osteotomies can be performed prone, supine, or in the lateral decubitus position based on surgeon preference and typically involve the use of a blade plate, locking plate, or an IM nail. Intertrochanteric plate-stabilized osteotomies begin with a proximal/lateral incision centered over the greater trochanter. The fascia lata is split to expose the insertion of the gluteus medius and the origin of the vastus lateralis. A transgluteal or vastus elevating approach can be used followed by an anterior capsulotomy. If a blade plate is being used, a cortical window is made and the U-shaped chisel is introduced. Two K wires are placed anterior to posterior to allow for rotational measurements and the osteotomy is completed perpendicular to the long axis of the femur. A broad chisel is used to open the osteotomy and the chisel and the patient's foot are used as levers to manipulate the fragments. The chisel is exchanged for a blade plate, rotational correction is verified, and the plate is affixed to both the proximal and distal fragments, while exercising care not to alter coronal or sagittal plane alignment. Depending on the mode of fixation, partial weight-bearing is typically maintained for 6 to 8 weeks.[63]

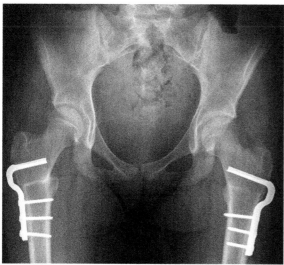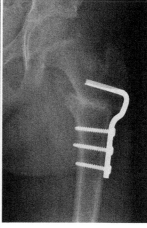

Fig. 6. An intertrochanteric osteotomy is fixed with a blade plate.

Diaphyseal femoral osteotomy

Diaphyseal osteotomies typically involve the use of an IM nail (**Fig. 7**). Benefits of this location and mode of fixation include immediate weight-bearing with the IM nail and the provisions for large corrections. Potential drawbacks include the need to make multiple incisions, the lack of control over coronal plane deformities, and slower bone healing which can average 3 to 4 months.[64] Buly and colleagues reported on the outcomes of 55 diaphyseal osteotomies over a period of 6.5 years.[64] Clinical improvement was demonstrated in the most of the patients with 75% reporting "excellent" results. One nonunion was reported and 39 of the implants were ultimately removed because of hardware irritation or thigh pain.[64]

Diaphyseal osteotomies are typically performed supine or in the lateral decubitus position based on surgeon preference. Separate approaches are made to the osteotomy site and nail entry site. Typically, a small skin incision can be made just proximal to the greater trochanter to allow access to the starting point for either a piriformis or trochanteric entry nail. If a retrograde nail is used, then the entry point is in the knee and can be done through the patellar tendon or adjacent to the patellar tendon. Once a nail diameter is selected, overreaming of the isthmus and subtrochanteric region by 0.5 mm is performed.[64] The placement of 2 Steinmann or Schanz pins, one proximal to the osteotomy and one proximal to the knee joint provides rotational alignment and control. The pin proximal to the knee joint can be placed with the patella pointing straight ahead to represent the frontal plane of the distal fragment.[59] It is important to keep these pins as posterior as possible to avoid conflict with the IM nail; particularly, the pin that is closest to the entry point of the IM canal. Next, the osteotomy is made using either an IM or extramedullary approach at the isthmus of

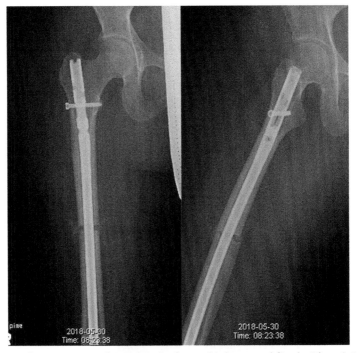

Fig. 7. Femoral osteotomy performed at the femoral isthmus and fixed with an intramedullary nail.

the canal, approximately one-third of the way moving in a proximal to distal direction.[59] IM cuts are made using a Winquist IM saw, which allows for a stepwise cut with progressive protrusion of the blade.[64] Alternatively, extramedullary cuts are made through a separate small incision and typically use a combination of drill bits, saws, and osteotomes. Extramedullary drilling, if performed before reaming, can allow for the added benefit of providing a route for reamings to extrude, hopefully reducing the risk of fat embolism.[57,59] Once the osteotomy is completed, the guide pin is advanced, gross rotational correction is completed, and the IM nail is introduced and locked on the entry side (either hip or knee) to the canal, via the guide. Final rotational adjustments are then made using the tibia as a handle to rotate the knee as opposed to using the reference pins which can become loose or dislodged.[59] Rotational correction is then confirmed using the reference pins or by the use of an external reference guide such as an inclinometer, and the interlocks are placed on the other end of the osteotomy from the IM entry.[59] Final hip range of motion is confirmed and incisions are closed. Postoperatively, the patient is typically weight-bearing as tolerated with crutches.

Distal femoral osteotomy

Distal osteotomies are typically performed in either the medial or lateral metaphyseal area and are commonly stabilized with a locking plate[57,58] (**Fig. 8**). Benefits of this location include a single incision for the osteotomy and fixation which can often be used for concomitant procedures about the knee and the ability to make coronal plane as well as axial plane corrections.[58] Potential disadvantages would include a higher risk of neurovascular injury and a potentially more restrictive immediate postoperative weight-bearing or range of motion depending on the mode of fixation. Both medial and lateral distal femoral osteotomies have demonstrated good clinical outcomes.[65,66] Nelitz and colleagues reported on 16-month follow-up for 12 patients undergoing medial-sided osteotomies and reported no-repeat patellar dislocations with a median IKDC score improving from 60 to 85. Two patients did demonstrate a slight (10°) flexion deficit without subjective impairment.[66] Laterally based osteotomies have demonstrated similarly excellent results. Imhoff and colleagues published results on 39 patients who followed up for 44 months and reported significant pain relief and clinical improvement, with no-repeat patella dislocations.[65] Plate removal was reported in

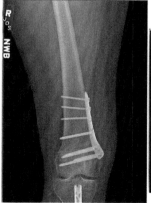
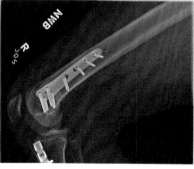

Fig. 8. Femoral osteotomy performed at the distal femur and fixed with a locking plate and screws. Coronal plane abnormalities can be addressed through this approach as well.

31 patients and at a mean 4-year follow-up, 72% of the patients were either very satisfied (n = 13) or satisfied (n = 15).[65]

Distal femoral osteotomies are performed in supine position using either a medial or lateral subvastus approach.[58,65,66] Laterally based incisions begin with a longitudinal split of the IT band. Subperiosteal dissection is performed and a blunt Hohmann retractor is used to protect the neurovascular structures behind the femoral shaft. Steinmann pins are then placed both proximal and distal to the planned osteotomy to judge rotation.[65,67] Using a combination of saws and osteotomes, osteotomy cuts are then completed. Osteotomy cuts perpendicular to the femoral shaft provide axial corrections, but oblique cuts can be used to allow for single osteotomy correction of both axial and coronal deformities.[68] Once the desired corrections have been verified, a locking distal femoral plate is used to provide fixation. Weight-bearing is typically partially restricted for up to 6 weeks with range of motion guidelines being dictated by concomitant procedures.[65,66]

Tibial Osteotomy

Initial questions to answer when performing a tibial osteotomy mirror those of a femoral osteotomy. Level of osteotomy and degree of correction must be determined, and whether to perform a fibular osteotomy must be decided. Similar to the femoral osteotomy, clear guiding evidence is lacking, so the best clinical judgment is used. Typical osteotomy sites include proximal "supratubercle" locations, diaphyseal, and more distal osteotomy sites.[69] Each location has advantages and disadvantages with planned corrections aimed at restoring a more normal thigh-foot axis. Interpreting the outcomes of these various osteotomies is challenging in that many of the reported patient populations include young patients with neuromuscular disorders, as opposed to more athletic populations.[69–73]

Proximal tibial osteotomy

Proximal osteotomies are performed proximal to the tibial tubercle with one benefit being the ability to provide correction of both axial and coronal plane deformities.[69] If increased tibial tubercle trochlear groove (TTTG) distances are present, computer modeling has shown a 0.68 mm reduction in TTTG distances per degree of derotation performed in a proximal fashion.[71] One must be cognizant of where the rotational deformity lies, however, as with external tibial torsions of more than 35°; a large portion of the deformity can be distal to the tibial tubercle.[74] Other potential advantages include secondary compression from the extensor mechanism as well as a large metaphyseal area of bone contact for healing.[69] Potential disadvantages include the concern for peroneal nerve injury, compartment syndrome, and potentially more challenging fixation techniques. This has led to recommendations that supratubercle osteotomies be performed only for small corrections, typically less than 15°. Dickschas reported on the outcomes of 49 proximal tibial osteotomies with an average correction of 10.8°.[70] The authors also showed correction of coronal deformity in 21 cases, with 7 of those requiring proximal fibular osteotomy.[70] They reported one nonunion that underwent revision fixation with bone grafting, and one painful fibular pseudoarthrosis was reported.[70] They also documented one compartment syndrome requiring acute compartment release as well as a transient peroneal nerve palsy.[70] Krengel and Staheli demonstrated a 13% complication rate for their proximal osteotomies, including compartment syndrome, peroneal nerve palsy, and a deep infection.[75] These findings led the authors to recommend distal osteotomies in which their serious complication rate was zero.[75]

Proximal tibial osteotomies are typically performed supine and use a lateral approach. A lateral incision allows for access to both the tibia and fibula, as well as the lateral retinaculum.[70] The anterior muscle compartment is released from the proximal tibia and the planned osteotomy site is identified.[70] Pins are placed to allow for measurement of rotation and either a single or biplanar osteotomy is performed based on the inclusion of the tibial tubercle. A maximum of 20° torsional correction is recommended, with any corrections greater than 12°, likely requiring a neurolysis of the peroneal nerve.[70] Stabilization can be provided by locking or nonlocking plates with immediate range of motion and partial weight-bearing for 6 weeks.[70]

Diaphyseal tibial osteotomy

Diaphyseal osteotomies are typically performed in the cortical midshaft area (**Fig. 9**). These osteotomies are generally limited to correction of axial plane deformities and use an IM nail, although there is some ability to correct coronal plane deformity if the osteotomy is completed in the proximal metadiaphyseal area.[72] Diaphyseal and more distal osteotomies are perceived to be technically easier and safer with regard to injury to the neurovascular structures.[69] Other benefits of IM fixation include early load sharing of the implant, less soft tissue disruption at the osteotomy site, and early weight-bearing.[73] The primary disadvantage is the delayed healing often seen in a diaphyseal osteotomy. Stotts and Stevens performed 59 diaphyseal osteotomies, which were stabilized by IM nailing and reported an 8.5% major complication rate.[73] Their average correction was 28.8° with a fibular osteotomy being performed in the first patient but was not felt to be needed subsequently.[73] Nearly, all patients

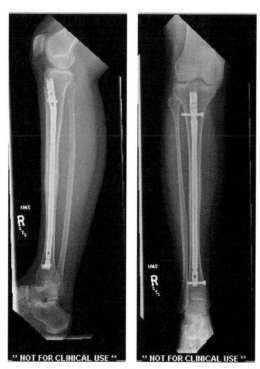

Fig. 9. Tibial osteotomy performed at the tibial isthmus and fixed with an intramedullary nail.

underwent prophylactic anterior compartment fasciotomy releases and 85% of the IM nails were removed. At final follow-up (22.6 months), 76% of the patients reported no pain in the extremity.[73] Ferri-de-Barros reported on the outcomes of 20 diaphyseal osteotomies with an average correction of 33°.[76] Nineteen of the osteotomies healed without major complication, with a pseudoarthrosis developing in one patient that required a revision exchange nailing and fibular osteotomy.[76]

Diaphyseal osteotomies are typically performed supine on a radiolucent table similar to IM nailing for fractures.[76] A standard IM nailing incision and approach is used proximally. A prophylactic drill hole is then placed in the midshaft before reaming to help prevent fat emboli, followed by reaming of the IM canal and placement of Kirschner wires to allow for correction measurement.[76] The nail is then introduced over the guidewire up to the osteotomy site, followed by the creation of the osteotomy. This can be accomplished using several methods including multiple drill holes, sagittal saw, osteotomes, or a combination of methods. A concomitant prophylactic anterior compartment fasciotomy is typically performed at the time of surgery.[73,76] Proximal fixation is performed and then once the desired correction is obtained, distal interlocks are placed followed by a standard closure.[73,76] Weight-bearing and range of motion are typically not restricted with IM fixation.[76]

Distal tibial osteotomy

Distal osteotomies are performed in the metaphyseal area of the distal tibia and can be stabilized with a plate and screw construct[77] or by using an external fixator[78] (**Fig. 10**). Benefits of this location include a wider metaphyseal contact area for bony healing as

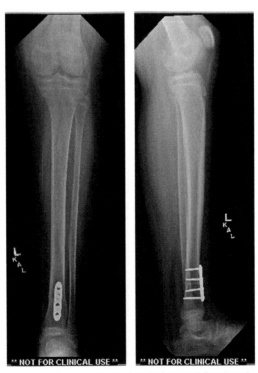

Fig. 10. Tibial osteotomy performed at the distal tibia and fixed with a plate and screws. Note that the plate is placed proximal to the distal tibial physis.

well as a reduced incidence of neuromuscular injury.[69] Drawbacks include the need for more restrictive postoperative weight-bearing. Selber and colleagues performed 91 supramalleolar osteotomies and reported a 5.3% incidence of major complications (nonunion [n = 1], osteotomy site fracture [n = 1], distal tibia growth arrest [n = 1]).[77] Distal fibula osteotomies were also performed in all patients with an average correction of 26°.[69-73] Erschbamer and colleagues performed a more proximal metadiaphyseal osteotomy and used an external fixator to provide stability in a series of 71 osteotomies.[78] Concomitant fibular osteotomy was performed only if planned correction exceeded 30° (n = 8). All patients obtained eventual healing with removal of the external fixator at a mean of 104 days.[78] Two patients did experience fractures after removal of the external fixator but were subsequently treated and went on to union.[78] No other serious complications were reported.[78]

Distal osteotomies are typically performed supine on a radiolucent table and typically use an anterior approach to the distal tibia.[77,78] Once the osteotomy site is identified, proximal and distal pins are placed to allow for rotational corrections with care being exercised not to injure the tibialis anterior tendon. The osteotomy is then completed using drill pins, gigli or sagittal saw, or osteotomes, followed by rotational corrections, and finally, stabilization with either a plate/screw or external fixator construct.[77,78] Weight-bearing and range of motion are typically dictated by the mode of fixation.

The need for a fibular osteotomy

There is debate on the indications for inclusion of a concomitant fibular osteotomy when performing a tibial osteotomy.[69] Proponents argue that the additional fibular osteotomy reduces the tension at the tibial osteotomy site, facilitating easier and larger corrections. Most authors reported using a fibular osteotomy when full corrections could not be achieved, or prophylactically when larger corrections were anticipated and have been reported more often in the literature with proximal or distal osteotomies as opposed to diaphyseal locations.[69,73,76,77]

SURGICAL INDICATIONS

As indicated from the available literature, there are not yet clear guidelines on surgical indications. Currently, the surgical algorithm for the authors is based on groupings of 10° of axial plane abnormality. 0° to 20° is within a normal range and not corrected surgically. 20° to 30° may be abnormal but would only lead to surgery if there was further evidence such as gait analysis demonstrating that the axial plane abnormality may be contributing to PF pathology. 30° to 40° is concerning and sometimes leads to surgical correction, but is considered in the setting of other PF anatomic risk factors. Above 40° almost always leads to surgical correction. This approach is used for both femur and tibia. If the femur range is not concerning, then only the tibia is addressed. If the femur is concerning, then most often the tibia is also in a concerning range of axial plane rotation, and both the femur and tibia are correctly surgically at the same time. Occasionally, the femur has significant axial plane abnormality, but the tibia does not. In this setting, it is possible to address only the femur, but this decision should be based on examination and careful decision-making by the surgeon because the femoral derotation will externally rotate the distal femur such that the tibia is also externally rotated. It is also possible to correct either femur or tibia more than the other to better align both the femur and the tibia.

SUMMARY

Rotational deformity is a less common cause of patellar instability than trochlear dysplasia and patella alta, but is an important risk factor for any PF surgeon to consider. In some cases, rotational deformity is the primary bony factor producing the instability and should be corrected surgically. More research is needed on what are normal values for femoral version and tibial torsion, as well as when the axial plane alignment needs to be corrected, but this is a growing area of study. There are many tools that can be used to evaluate the axial plane and surgeons should be familiar with each of them. Understanding the advantages and disadvantages of each site for osteotomy will help the surgeon choose the most appropriate osteotomy depending on patient anatomy and skeletal maturity status.

CLINICS CARE POINTS

- Femoral version and tibial torsion are risk factors for patellofemoral instability because they cause excessive rotation of the patellofemoral joint during dynamic motion.
- For patients with patellofemoral instability, gather a thorough history including any history that may suggest rotational deformity.
- Be sure to include a rotational evaluation as part of the physical examination.
- Understand the various diagnostic tools for evaluating rotational deformity in patients with patellofemoral instability, and do not hesitate to use more than one to inform confidence in the findings before deciding on surgery.
- Understand the advantages and disadvantages of derotation osteotomy at each level to choose the appropriate surgery for individual patients.

DISCLOSURE

Dr E.A. Arendt is a paid consultant and educational speaker for Smith & Nephew. The other authors have nothing to disclose.

REFERENCES

1. Ries Z, Bollier M. Patellofemoral Instability in Active Adolescents. J Knee Surg 2015;28(4):265–77.
2. le Damany PG. Technique of tibial tropometry. Clin Orthop Relat Res 1903; 1994(302):4–10 [discussion: 12–3].
3. Eckhoff DG, Johnson KK. Three-dimensional computed tomography reconstruction of tibial torsion. Clin Orthop Relat Res 1994;(302):42–6.
4. Elfman H. Torsion of the lower extremity. Am J Phys Anthropol 1945;3(3):255–65.
5. Hutter CG Jr, Scott W. Tibial torsion. J Bone Joint Surg Am 1949;31a(3):511–8.
6. Yoshioka Y, Siu DW, Scudamore RA, et al. Tibial anatomy and functional axes. J Orthop Res 1989;7(1):132–7.
7. Lincoln TL, Suen PW. Common rotational variations in children. J Am Acad Orthop Surg 2003;11(5):312–20.
8. Kristiansen LP, Gunderson RB, Steen H, et al. The normal development of tibial torsion. Skeletal Radiol 2001;30(9):519–22.
9. Scorcelletti M, Reeves ND, Rittweger J, et al. Femoral anteversion: significance and measurement. J Anat 2020;237(5):811–26.
10. Botser IB, Ozoude GC, Martin DE, et al. Femoral anteversion in the hip: comparison of measurement by computed tomography, magnetic resonance imaging, and physical examination. Arthroscopy 2012;28(5):619–27.

11. Staheli L. Rotational Problems in Children. J Bone Joint Surgery-American Volume 75a 1993;6:939–52.
12. Salsich GB, Perman WH. Patellofemoral joint contact area is influenced by tibio-femoral rotation alignment in individuals who have patellofemoral pain. J Orthop Sports Phys Ther 2007;37(9):521–8.
13. Lee TQ, Morris G, Csintalan RP. The influence of tibial and femoral rotation on pa-tellofemoral contact area and pressure. J Orthop Sports Phys Ther 2003;33(11):686–93.
14. Souza RB, Draper CE, Fredericson M, et al. Femur rotation and patellofemoral joint kinematics: a weight-bearing magnetic resonance imaging analysis. J Orthop Sports Phys Ther 2010;40(5):277–85.
15. Kaiser P, Schmoelz W, Schoettle P, et al. Increased internal femoral torsion can be regarded as a risk factor for patellar instability - A biomechanical study. Clin Bio-mech (Bristol, Avon) 2017;47:103–9.
16. Powers CM. The influence of altered lower-extremity kinematics on patellofemoral joint dysfunction: a theoretical perspective. J Orthop Sports Phys Ther 2003;33(11):639–46.
17. Paulos L, Swanson SC, Stoddard GJ, et al. Surgical correction of limb malalign-ment for instability of the patella: a comparison of 2 techniques. Am J Sports Med 2009;37(7):1288–300.
18. Aiona M, Calligeros K, Pierce R. Coronal plane knee moments improve after cor-recting external tibial torsion in patients with cerebral palsy. Clin Orthop Relat Res 2012;470(5):1327–33.
19. Turner MS. The association between tibial torsion and knee joint pathology. Clin Orthop Relat Res 1994;(302):47–51.
20. Schwartz M, Lakin G. The effect of tibial torsion on the dynamic function of the soleus during gait. Gait Posture 2003;17(2):113–8.
21. Chung CY, Lee KM, Park MS, et al. Validity and reliability of measuring femoral anteversion and neck-shaft angle in patients with cerebral palsy. J Bone Joint Surg Am 2010;92(5):1195–205.
22. Lee SH, Chung CY, Park MS, et al. Tibial torsion in cerebral palsy: validity and reliability of measurement. Clin Orthop Relat Res 2009;467(8):2098–104.
23. Martin HD, Palmer IJ. History and physical examination of the hip: the basics. Curr Rev Musculoskelet Med 2013;6(3):219–25.
24. Ruwe PA, Gage JR, Ozonoff MB, et al. Clinical determination of femoral antever-sion. A comparison with established techniques. J Bone Joint Surg Am 1992;74(6):820–30.
25. Staheli LT, Corbett M, Wyss C, et al. Lower-extremity rotational problems in chil-dren. Normal values to guide management. J Bone Joint Surg Am 1985;67(1):39–47.
26. Gage J, Schwartz M, Koop S, et al. The identification and treatment of gait prob-lems in cerebral palsy. 2nd edition. Hoboken, NJ: Press MK; 2009.
27. Staheli LT, Engel GM. Tibial torsion: a method of assessment and a survey of normal children. Clin Orthop Relat Res 1972;86:183–6.
28. Shih YC, Chau MM, Arendt EA, et al. Measuring Lower Extremity Rotational Align-ment: A Review of Methods and Case Studies of Clinical Applications. J Bone Joint Surg Am 2020;102(4):343–56.
29. Dunlap K, Shands AR Jr, Hollister LC Jr, et al. A new method for determination of torsion of the femur. J Bone Joint Surg Am 1953;35-a(2):289–311.
30. Kingsley PC, Olmsted KL. A study to determine the angle of anteversion of the neck of the femur. J Bone Joint Surg Am 1948;30a(3):745–51.

31. Sugano N, Noble PC, Kamaric E. A comparison of alternative methods of measuring femoral anteversion. J Comput Assist Tomogr 1998;22(4):610–4.

32. Hernandez RJ, Tachdjian MO, Poznanski AK, et al. CT determination of femoral torsion. AJR Am J Roentgenol 1981;137(1):97–101.

33. Kaiser P, Attal R, Kammerer M, et al. Significant differences in femoral torsion values depending on the CT measurement technique. Arch Orthop Trauma Surg 2016;136(9):1259–64.

34. Schmaranzer F, Lerch TD, Siebenrock KA, et al. Differences in Femoral Torsion Among Various Measurement Methods Increase in Hips With Excessive Femoral Torsion. Clin Orthop Relat Res 2019;477(5):1073–83.

35. Schneider B, Laubenberger J, Jemlich S, et al. Measurement of femoral antetorsion and tibial torsion by magnetic resonance imaging. Br J Radiol 1997;70(834): 575–9.

36. Beebe MJ, Wylie JD, Bodine BG, et al. Accuracy and Reliability of Computed Tomography and Magnetic Resonance Imaging Compared With True Anatomic Femoral Version. J Pediatr Orthop 2017;37(4):e265–70.

37. Hesham K, Carry PM, Freese K, et al. Measurement of Femoral Version by MRI is as Reliable and Reproducible as CT in Children and Adolescents With Hip Disorders. J Pediatr Orthop 2017;37(8):557–62.

38. Muhamad AR, Freitas JM, Bomar JD, et al. CT and MRI lower extremity torsional profile studies: measurement reproducibility. J Child Orthop 2012;6(5):391–6.

39. Tomczak RJ, Guenther KP, Rieber A, et al. MR imaging measurement of the femoral antetorsional angle as a new technique: comparison with CT in children and adults. AJR Am J Roentgenol 1997;168(3):791–4.

40. Chaibi Y, Cresson T, Aubert B, et al. Fast 3D reconstruction of the lower limb using a parametric model and statistical inferences and clinical measurements calculation from biplanar X-rays. Comput Methods Biomech Biomed Engin 2012;15(5): 457–66.

41. Buck FM, Guggenberger R, Koch PP, et al. Femoral and tibial torsion measurements with 3D models based on low-dose biplanar radiographs in comparison with standard CT measurements. AJR Am J Roentgenol 2012;199(5):W607–12.

42. Folinais D, Thelen P, Delin C, et al. Measuring femoral and rotational alignment: EOS system versus computed tomography. Orthop Traumatol Surg Res 2013; 99(5):509–16.

43. Gaumétou E, Quijano S, Ilharreborde B, et al. EOS analysis of lower extremity segmental torsion in children and young adults. Orthop Traumatol Surg Res 2014;100(1):147–51.

44. Meyrignac O, Moreno R, Baunin C, et al. Low-dose biplanar radiography can be used in children and adolescents to accurately assess femoral and tibial torsion and greatly reduce irradiation. Eur Radiol 2015;25(6):1752–60.

45. Pomerantz ML, Glaser D, Doan J, et al. Three-dimensional biplanar radiography as a new means of accessing femoral version: a comparitive study of EOS three-dimensional radiography versus computed tomography. Skeletal Radiol 2015; 44(2):255–60.

46. Rosskopf AB, Buck FM, Pfirrmann CW, et al. Femoral and tibial torsion measurements in children and adolescents: comparison of MRI and 3D models based on low-dose biplanar radiographs. Skeletal Radiol 2017;46(4):469–76.

47. Rosskopf AB, Ramseier LE, Sutter R, et al. Femoral and tibial torsion measurement in children and adolescents: comparison of 3D models based on low-dose biplanar radiography and low-dose CT. AJR Am J Roentgenol 2014; 202(3):W285–91.

48. Blumer SL, Dinan D, Grissom LE. Benefits and unexpected artifacts of biplanar digital slot-scanning imaging in children. Pediatr Radiol 2014;44(7):871–82.
49. Hull PD, Johnson SC, Stephen DJ, et al. Delayed debridement of severe open fractures is associated with a higher rate of deep infection. Bone Joint J 2014; 96-b(3):379–84.
50. Melhem E, Assi A, El Rachkidi R, et al. EOS(®) biplanar X-ray imaging: concept, developments, benefits, and limitations. J Child Orthop 2016;10(1):1–14.
51. Davis RB, Ounpuu S, Tyburski D, et al. A gait analysis data collection and reduction technique. Hum Mov Sci 1991;10(5):575–87.
52. Schwartz MH, Rozumalski A. A new method for estimating joint parameters from motion data. J Biomech 2005;38(1):107–16.
53. Radler C, Kranzl A, Manner HM, et al. Torsional profile versus gait analysis: consistency between the anatomic torsion and the resulting gait pattern in patients with rotational malalignment of the lower extremity. Gait Posture 2010;32(3):405–10.
54. Tornetta P 3rd, Ritz G, Kantor A. Femoral torsion after interlocked nailing of unstable femoral fractures. J Trauma 1995;38(2):213–9.
55. Yang KH, Han DY, Jahng JS, et al. Prevention of malrotation deformity in femoral shaft fracture. J Orthop Trauma 1998;12(8):558–62.
56. Clementz BG. Assessment of tibial torsion and rotational deformity with a new fluoroscopic technique. Clin Orthop Relat Res 1989;(245):199–209.
57. Nelitz M. Femoral Derotational Osteotomies. Curr Rev Musculoskelet Med 2018; 11(2):272–9.
58. Biedert RM. Reflections on Rotational Osteotomies around the Patellofemoral Joint. J Clin Med 2021;10(3).
59. Steiebel M, Paley D. Derotational Osteotomies of the Femur and Tibia for Recurrent Patellar Instability. Oper Tech Sports Med 2019;27(4):1–8.
60. Edmonds EW, Fuller CB, Jeffords ME, et al. Femoral derotational osteotomy level does not effect resulting torsion. J Exp Orthop 2020;7(1):9.
61. Sung KH, Kwon SS, Chung CY, et al. Long-term outcomes over 10 years after femoral derotation osteotomy in ambulatory children with cerebral palsy. Gait Posture 2018;64:119–25.
62. Hatem M, Khoury AN, Erickson LR, et al. Femoral Derotation Osteotomy Improves Hip and Spine Function in Patients With Increased or Decreased Femoral Torsion. Arthroscopy 2021;37(1):111–23.
63. Ledezma C, Henle P, Tannast M, et al. Proximal femoral osteotomy. 2nd edition. Philadelphia: Lippincott Williams and Wilkins; 2015.
64. Buly RL, Sosa BR, Poultsides LA, et al. Femoral Derotation Osteotomy in Adults for Version Abnormalities. J Am Acad Orthop Surg 2018;26(19):e416–25.
65. Imhoff FB, Cotic M, Liska F, et al. Derotational osteotomy at the distal femur is effective to treat patients with patellar instability. Knee Surg Sports Traumatol Arthrosc 2019;27(2):652–8.
66. Nelitz M, Dreyhaupt J, Williams SR, et al. Combined supracondylar femoral derotation osteotomy and patellofemoral ligament reconstruction for recurrent patellar dislocation and severe femoral anteversion syndrome: surgical technique and clinical outcome. Int Orthop 2015;39(12):2355–62.
67. Zhang Z, Zhang H, Song G, et al. A High-Grade J Sign Is More Likely to Yield Higher Postoperative Patellar Laxity and Residual Maltracking in Patients With Recurrent Patellar Dislocation Treated With Derotational Distal Femoral Osteotomy. Am J Sports Med 2020;48(1):117–27.

68. Imhoff FB, Schnell J, Magaña A, et al. Single cut distal femoral osteotomy for correction of femoral torsion and valgus malformity in patellofemoral malalignment - proof of application of new trigonometrical calculations and 3D-printed cutting guides. BMC Musculoskelet Disord 2018;19(1):215.

69. Snow M. Tibial Torsion and Patellofemoral Pain and Instability in the Adult Population: Current Concept Review. Curr Rev Musculoskelet Med 2021;14(1):67–75.

70. Dickschas J, Tassika A, Lutter C, et al. Torsional osteotomies of the tibia in patellofemoral dysbalance. Arch Orthop Trauma Surg 2017;137(2):179–85.

71. Jud L, Singh S, Tondelli T, et al. Combined Correction of Tibial Torsion and Tibial Tuberosity-Trochlear Groove Distance by Supratuberositary Torsional Osteotomy of the Tibia. Am J Sports Med 2020;48(9):2260–7.

72. Kim KI, Thaller PH, Ramteke A, et al. Corrective tibial osteotomy in young adults using an intramedullary nail. Knee Surg Relat Res 2014;26(2):88–96.

73. Stotts AK, Stevens PM. Tibial rotational osteotomy with intramedullary nail fixation. Strateg Trauma Limb Reconstr 2009;4(3):129–33.

74. Winkler PW, Lutz PM, Rupp MC, et al. Increased external tibial torsion is an infratuberositary deformity and is not correlated with a lateralized position of the tibial tuberosity. Knee Surg Sports Traumatol Arthrosc 2021;29(5):1678–85.

75. Krengel WF 3rd, Staheli LT. Tibial rotational osteotomy for idiopathic torsion. A comparison of the proximal and distal osteotomy levels. Clin Orthop Relat Res 1992;283:285–9.

76. Ferri-de-Barros F, Inan M, Miller F. Intramedullary nail fixation of femoral and tibial percutaneous rotational osteotomy in skeletally mature adolescents with cerebral palsy. J Pediatr Orthop 2006;26(1):115–8.

77. Selber P, Filho ER, Dallalana R, et al. Supramalleolar derotation osteotomy of the tibia, with T plate fixation. Technique and results in patients with neuromuscular disease. J Bone Joint Surg Br 2004;86(8):1170–5.

78. Erschbamer M, Gerhard P, Klima H, et al. Distal tibial derotational osteotomy with external fixation to treat torsional deformities: a review of 71 cases. J Pediatr Orthop B 2017;26(2):179–83.

Genu Valgum Correction and Biplanar Osteotomies

Scott Taylor, MBBS(Hons), BMedSc, FRACS(Orth), FAOrthA, Alan Getgood, MPhil MD FRCS(Tr&Orth)*

KEYWORDS

- Patellofemoral instability • Valgus malalignment • Osteotomy
- Distal femoral osteotomy (DFO) • High tibial osteotomy (HTO)

KEY POINTS

- Correction of valgus coronal plane malalignment should be considered when assessing patients with patella instability.
- Correction should be tailored to the individual patient's anatomy and can be performed on the femur, tibia, or in rare cases both bones.
- On the femoral side, both medial closing and lateral opening wedge osteotomes are viable and effective treatment options with equivalent complication profiles despite their theoretic differences.
- Osteotomy is most often combined with a soft tissue procedure and results in reliable reduction in patient symptoms.

INTRODUCTION

Genu valgum is a potential contributor to patellofemoral instability.[1–3] With increasing amounts of valgus angulation, the Q angle increases, resulting in a lateralizing force vector on the patella with respect to the trochlear groove.[4] Correcting valgus angulation has multiple possible advantages. Importantly, neutralizing the valgus reduces this lateral force vector by effectively medializing the tibial tuberosity and thus decreases the risk of recurrent dislocation.[5–7] It may also prevent the advancement or development of osteoarthritis in both the lateral tibiofemoral and patellofemoral compartment, although this has not been studied long-term in the patellar dislocation population.[8–10] Last, it may also improve subjective sense of knee stability due to reduction of the abduction moment during stance phase.[11] Despite the intuitive relationship between genu valgum and patella instability, evidence on the effectiveness of correction is limited to case series and reports,[1,2,4,11] making definitive statements about its clinical utility challenging.

Department of Surgery, Fowler Kennedy Sports Medicine Clinic, Western University, London, Ontario, Canada
* Corresponding author.
E-mail address: alan.getgood@uwo.ca

Clin Sports Med 41 (2022) 47–63
https://doi.org/10.1016/j.csm.2021.08.001
0278-5919/22/© 2021 Elsevier Inc. All rights reserved.

CLINICAL INDICATIONS

Indications for correction of coronal plane valgus alignment include symptomatic patella instability. Definitions of patella instability vary in the literature; however, patients with recurrent dislocation, subluxations, and habitual dislocation have all been successfully treated with the procedure.[4,9,12–14] Particular attention must be paid to the presence of untreated valgus in the setting of revision surgery; however, the threshold for intervention in the primary setting is unclear. A minimum threshold of mechanical tibiofemoral angle (mTFA) of 5° to 6° of valgus has been described with good results,[15,16] although values as low as 2° also have been used.[9] There are no studies that clearly define a degree of valgus, over which provides optimal outcome. As such, a careful examination of all bony and soft tissue factors contributing to the individual patient's instability presents multiple opportunities for intervention. Identifying those at highest priority for intervention is challenging. Successful outcomes con be achieved through coronal plane correction alone[14]; however, most studies involve osteotomy in combination with at least one other procedure. Soft tissue procedures, such as medial reefing, lateral release,[1,2,4,9,12,15,16] and medial patellofemoral ligament (MPFL) reconstruction,[1] as well as bony procedures such as tibial tubercle osteotomy and derotational osteotomies[4] have all been described. The presence of combined femoral anteversion and valgus may be treated together in a single supracondylar femoral osteotomy.[17,18] Swarup and colleagues[4] articulated "symptomatic" genu valgum, valgus in the presence of lateral knee pain, as the threshold for coronal plane correction. However, many patients with patella instability do not present with pain and thus other factors such as magnitude of valgus, ligamentous laxity, or absence of other correctable risk factors may be indications to proceed with osteotomy.[12,13]

Contraindications to coronal plane correction must also be considered. Certainly, medial compartment osteoarthritis is a contraindication for valgus correction but is fortunately rare in the patellofemoral instability population. Similarly, patellofemoral degenerative change has also been described as a contraindication[15]; however, both trochlear and patella-sided chondral injuries have been shown to improve following distal femoral osteotomy.[9] As with most osteotomies, additional consideration must be given when offering surgery to patients with high body mass index and regular nicotine users.[12]

CLINICAL ASSESSMENT

Assessment involves that outlined in the article by Davis L Rogers and Andrew J. Cosgarea's article, "Evaluating Patellofemoral Patients: Physical Examination, Radiographic Imaging, and Measurements," elsewhere in this issue, with special attention to certain areas. The identification of valgus centers on visual inspection of standing coronal plane alignment and thus the clinician should have a low clinical threshold for obtaining radiographic assessment. The patient is assessed for both static and dynamic indicators of patella maltracking. The Q angle should be measured, with higher Q angles indicating an increased lateral subluxation vector on the patella.[19] Care must be taken not to confuse a high Q angle with lateral patella tracking, as high Q angles are more commonly associated with medial rather than lateral patella placement.[20] Regardless, patients with genu valgum will have increased Q angles and correction of the valgus medializes the tibial tubercle and will normalize the Q angle.[18]

The patient is carefully assessed for a J-sign in terminal extension/early flexion. Although the assessment is subjective, it clearly indicates excessive lateral patella translation in terminal extension.[20] The severity of the J-sign can often be better appreciated when the leg moves from the extended to flexed position, as the patella may often "jump" back into the groove from its more lateralized position. The exact cause is not fully known, but may be a reflection of coronal or rotational deformities, patella alta, trochlear dysplasia, and muscle imbalance.[21] Regardless of cause, the presence of a J-sign may indicate a more complex deformity and be associated with increased risk of isolated MPFL reconstruction failure.[22]

Identification of associated rotational deformities, increased femoral anteversion, and tibial torsion are made initially by assessing for squinting patella and in-toeing during gait and quantified further using hip range of motion and foot thigh angle in the prone position.

RADIOGRAPHIC ASSESSMENT

Long leg alignment films are taken. The mechanical axis of the limb is visualized by drawing a vertical line from the center of the femoral head to the center of the talus (**Fig. 1**).[23] Valgus is noted if the line passes lateral to the tibial spines and can be quantified by measuring the mTFA (Normal = $-1.0 \pm 2.8°$).[24] The site of deformity is identified by measurement of the anatomic lateral distal femoral angle (aLDFA; Normal = $81° \pm 2°$) as well as the medial proximal tibial angle (mPTA; Normal = $87° \pm 2°$) noting that there may be deformity at more than 1 level (**Fig. 2**).[20]

Careful attention should be paid to the positioning of the limb in the alignment radiograph. It is common to have these films taken with the patella pointing forward. In the patella instability population, the patella often sits more laterally. Thus, when the patellae are positioned forward, the femur may be internally rotated. This can result in the appearance of a valgus deformity, particularly if there are coexisting torsional abnormalities. A repeat alignment radiograph should be performed with the beam centered on getting an anteroposterior view of the knee. A clinical examination will help further determine whether torsional abnormalities coexist.

DECISION-MAKING ALGORITHM

See **Fig. 3** for the decision-making algorithm:

- What is the site of pathology?
  ○ Distal femur versus proximal tibia or both
- Does the size of correction warrant consideration of a double level osteotomy?
- How to correct?
  ○ Opening versus closing osteotomy?

FEMUR VERSUS TIBIA

The site of deformity and size of correction are the 2 main factors traditionally considered in selecting the level of osteotomy. For congenital valgus, the deformity is most often encountered in the distal femur and is addressed at that site. For tibial-sided deformities, size of correction is important due to the joint line obliquity created during the osteotomy. Significant joint line obliquity may result in progressive lateral subluxation of the tibia.[25] Therefore, patients with total valgus of 12° or post osteotomy proximal tibial joint line obliquity greater than 10° are likely better treated with femoral-sided osteotomy.[6,26] In the osteoarthritis literature, secondary consideration is given to the fact that tibial-sided osteotomy maintains correction throughout the range of motion.[27] Femoral osteotomy only corrects alignment in extension because at 90° of flexion the femoral weight-bearing surface moves to the posterior condyles: the position of which has not been changed by the coronal plane osteotomy.[28] The clinical relevance of this in patellofemoral instability has not yet been established.[22]

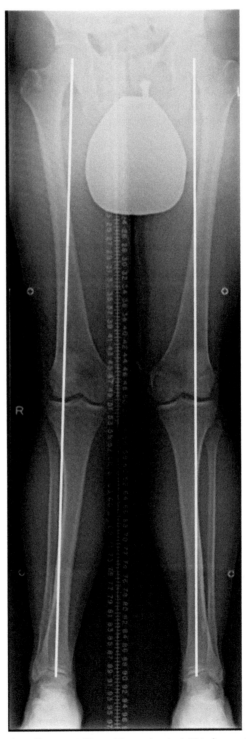

Fig. 1. Standing long leg alignment film with mechanical tibiofemoral angle displayed.

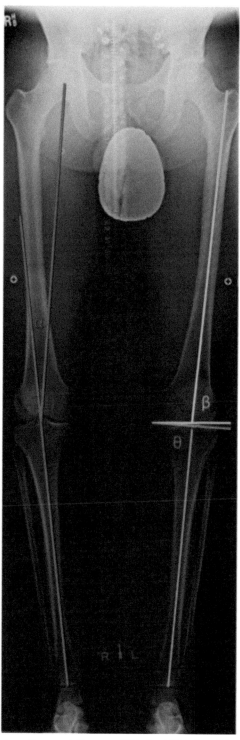

Fig. 2. Standing long leg alignment film. α: mTFA. β: aLDFA. θ: mPTA.

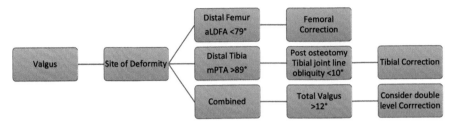

Fig. 3. Surgical decision-making algorithm.

Double-sided osteotomy can be considered when deformity at both the distal femur and proximal tibial is present[7,29] or in patients with significant valgus (mTFA >10°).[30] This allows for correction of both the joint line obliquity and coronal deformity.[30–32]

DISTAL FEMORAL MEDIAL CLOSING VERSUS LATERAL OPENING

In the following are considerations for the selection of opening versus closing wedge osteotomies of the femur (**Table 1**). In the osteoarthritis population, 2 systematic reviews described no difference in union or reoperation rates between the 2 techniques.[33–35] However, small numbers and study heterogeneity prevented rigorous statistical comparison rendering the choice to be one of personal preference.[26,27]

BIPLANAR OSTEOTOMIES IN CORONAL PLANE CORRECTION

There are many possible advantages for consideration of performing a biplanar osteotomy or biplanar "cuts." Biplanar osteotomies increase both axial stability of the osteotomy and increase the cancellous surface area for bone healing.[18,36–38] On the femoral side, the addition of an anterior cut in the coronal plane also allows for more distal positioning of the axial portion of the osteotomy, avoiding violation of the trochlea.[7] Furthermore, removal of a wedge of bone from the coronal plane osteotomy also allows for correction of axial/rotational deformities to be built into the osteotomy.[7,18,37,38] Biplanar correction can alternately be achieved by performing a single oblique osteotomy.[39]

CLINICAL OUTCOMES

Rigorous and long-term outcomes for valgus correction in the setting of patella instability is lacking in the literature. A recent systematic review by Tan and colleagues[40] analyzing femoral-sided corrections, included only 5 articles totaling 73 patients,[4,9,12–14] with significant heterogeneity preventing data pooling. Nevertheless, both radiologic and clinical outcomes reported at a mean of 4 years postoperatively are promising. All included studies demonstrated a radiologic improvement in joint alignment, measured either by mTFA or mLDFA. Postoperative instability was present in only 2 of the 73 patients. Interestingly, both patients came from an article studying the role of osteotomy alone, which highlights the possible benefits of concomitant soft tissue reconstruction in reducing this complication further. One patient had a subluxation event without effusion and declined further intervention, and the second underwent tibial tubercle osteotomy at 3 years post valgus correction.[14] Patient-reported outcome measures data vary widely; however, all studies reported an improvement in Kujala score. A clinically significant improvement in visual analog scale was noted in 3 studies.[4,9,13]

Table 1
Considerations for the selection of opening versus closing wedge osteotomies of the femur

Consideration	Opening Wedge	Closing Wedge
Approach	Femoral lateral approach is familiar and extensile	Femoral medial approach is limited proximally by neurovascular structures
Hardware prominence	More likely as irritates iliotibial band	Less likely
Correction titration	Fine tuning of correction possible through graduated wedge opening	Fine tuning difficult due to inherent challenge of bone wedge removal
Osteotomy stability	Less stable	Cortical apposition provides inherent stability
Bone grafting	May be necessary especially in larger corrections	Not required
Hinge fracture	Medial hinge fracture is on compression side	Lateral hinge fracture unstable due to tension side location

Schematic of the planning according to Dugdale and colleagues.[41]

PREOPERATIVE PLANNING

The osteotomy is planned according to the method described by Dugdale and colleagues[41] (**Fig. 4**).

This method can be applied to both femoral and tibial osteotomies. Care should be taken not to overcorrect, particularly on the femoral side, as the correction angle is measured at the joint line but the correction is made more proximally at the metadiaphyseal junction.

- Planning of lateral opening wedge high tibial osteotomy
  ○ Typically done according to Dugdale and colleagues[41] (see **Fig. 4**).
  ○ aLDFA should be normal.
  ○ Resultant correction will not create a joint line obliquity greater than 10°.
- Planning of medial closing wedge distal femoral osteotomy (MCWDFO)
  ○ Typically done according to Dugdale and colleagues[41] (see **Fig. 4**).
  ○ Desired weight-bearing line between center of knee to tip of medial tibial spine.
  ○ No overcorrection to varus to avoid overload.

PREPARATION AND POSITIONING

- Supine position on radiolucent/carbon table
- Lateral post lateral to the proximal thigh as well as footrest to enable a position of 30° flexion
- Tourniquet around proximal thigh (300 mm Hg)
- C-arm/fluoroscopy with sterile draping for intraoperative controls
  ○ Position on the opposite side of the patient to the osteotomy site
- Single-shot antibiotics following individual protocol for bone surgery
- Tranexamic acid 1 g intravenous at induction

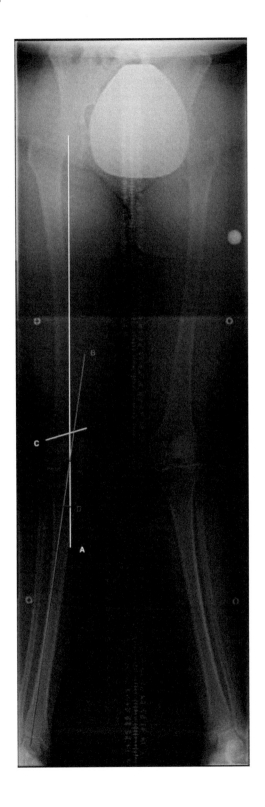

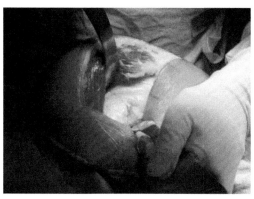

Fig. 5. Hohmann retractors in place over the anterior and posterior femoral cortices.

SURGICAL TECHNIQUE

The most commonly performed varus producing osteotomy in our practice is a medial closing wedge distal femoral osteotomy. This provides a very stable construct for early weight bearing and range of motion, with less likelihood for the need for hardware removal. The approach is on the medial side allowing for an easy approach to performing a concomitant MPFL reconstruction. Furthermore, in cases of recurrent lateral patella dislocation (LPD) in which the lateral retinacular structures are tight, a lateral opening wedge distal femoral osteotomy will cause and increase in lateral soft tissue tension, which can paradoxically make the LPD worse. It is common that an extensive lateral retinacular lengthening is required in these cases, and an MCWDFO does not compromise this soft tissue release.

- MCWDFO
  - ○ Medial skin incision
  - ○ The Epimysium over vastus medialis is incised and the muscle elevated off the medial intermuscular septum. The septum is then released off the periosteum. A cob elevator is used to elevate the posterior periosteum away from the posterior femoral cortex along the path of the planned osteotomy. A blunt Hohmann retractor is then placed on the anterior and posterior femoral cortices (**Fig. 5**).

◀───

Fig. 4. Calculation of osteotomy size. The planned mechanical axis is placed in the center of the tibia joint line from medial to lateral. Two lines are then drawn through this point. The first (*line A, white*) from the center of the femoral head and the second (*line B, red*) from the head of the talus. Ensure to extend these lines past the planned mechanical axis point. The intersection of these lines forms the angle of correction. To convert the angle of correction into millimeters of correction, the proposed osteotomy is drawn (*line C, green*), and the length of the line measured. From the planned mechanical axis point measure along line a, the distance of the proposed osteotomy. The distance from this point to line b is the millimeters of correction (*line D, blue*).[23,28] (*Data from* Puddu G, Cipolla M, Cerullo G, Franco V, Gianni, EG. Osteotomies: The Surgical Treatment of the Valgus Knee.; 2007., Chambat P, Selmi TAS, Dejour D, Denoyers J. Varus tibial osteotomy. Operative Techniques in Sports Medicine. 2000;8(1):44-47. doi:https://doi.org/10.1016/S1060-1872(00)80024-6)

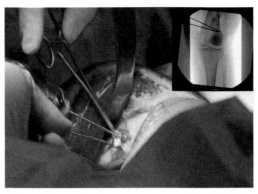

Fig. 6. Guide pin insertion using a ruler to ensure appropriate pin distance on medial cortex.

- o Guide pins are then inserted at the proximal and distal boundaries of the os-teotomy distanced at the medial cortex by the planned correction distance (**Fig. 6**). Their trajectory is checked with fluoroscopy. The length of the proximal and distal osteotomies is checked. Equal length will prevent a medial cortical step when the osteotomy is closed and impart stability to compression through cortical apposition.[37]
- o Mark the planned corticotomies with diathermy (**Fig. 7**). Biplanar femoral os-teotomy is performed with an oscillating saw starting with the distal osteotomy, then moving forward to the proximal osteotomy, completing both with an os-teotome to avoid lateral cortical breach. An additional coronal plane osteotomy is completed anteriorly providing rotational stability (**Fig. 8**), increased sur-faced area for union, and more straightforward removal of the wedge. The resultant wedge of bone is removed (**Fig. 9**). A punch can remove any residual posterior bone.
- o The osteotomy is closed gently and gradually to avoid hinge fractures. A controlled osteoclasis of the lateral hinge may be performed to weaken the cortical bridge without fracturing, using a 2.4-mm pin. The submuscular DFO locking plate is then positioned anteromedially on the distal femur. This

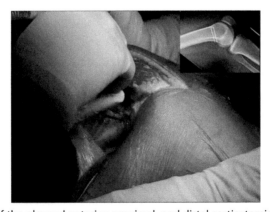

Fig. 7. Marking of the planned anterior, proximal, and distal corticotomies with diathermy. Inset: radiographic medial corticotomy plan.

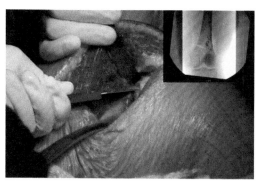

Fig. 8. Completion of the anterior or coronal plane osteotomy.

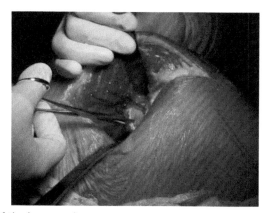

Fig. 9. Removal of the bone wedge.

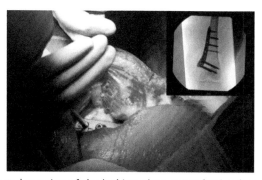

Fig. 10. Placement and securing of the locking plate. Inset: final radiographic appearance.

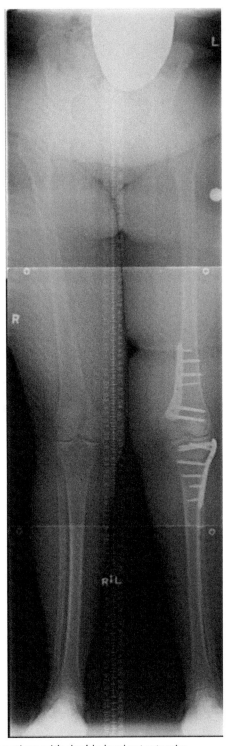

Fig. 11. Example of a patient with double level osteotomies.

Table 2
Complications specific to high tibial osteotomy and distal femoral osteotomy

Complication	Prevention	Correction
Intra-articular extension of osteotomy	• Ensure guide pin and subsequent osteotomy plane is ≥1 cm from articular surface • Do not open osteotomy until confirming anterior and posterior corticotomies are complete	• Confirm anterior corticotomies complete • Extend osteotomy with osteotome past extension before reattempting opening • If displaced consider reducing correction and fixing with screw before reattempting opening
Hinge fracture	• Ensure guide pin and subsequent osteotomy ends in meta-diaphysis not the diaphyseal cortical bone • Do not extend osteotomy within 1 cm of far cortex	• Consider fixation of osteotomy with locking plate • Use locking plate as reduction tool • Consider dual incision and fixation with staple if unable to address from operative side
Errors of correction	• Minimized by careful preoperative planning • Regular intraoperative radiograph use in both anteroposterior and lateral planes	• Adjustment of correction before application of definitive fixation
Neurovascular injury	• Familiarity with anatomy and approach • Limit proximal dissection in medial sub vastus approach • Maintain posterior refractors during instrumentation of the osteotomy	• Early identification aided by deflation of tourniquet before closure and close postoperative monitoring of neurovascular status
Hardware irritation	• Application of contoured plates in optimal anatomic location to avoid excess prominence • Consideration of medial femoral approach over lateral	• Hardware removal once osteotomy united
Delayed or malunion	• Preoperative patient optimization (eg, smoking cessation) • Consider grafting opening wedge osteotomies • Consider closing wedge osteotomies	• Exclusion of infection • Patient optimization • Revision in setting of loss of correction or impending hardware failure
Arthrofibrosis	• Stable osteotomy fixation allowing early range of motion and quads activation	• Manipulation under anesthesia • Arthroscopic arthrolysis

ensures the plate is positioned parallel with the femoral shaft proximally and has good coverage by the medial vastus to reduce mechanical irritation.
- ○ The plate is secured, and the closing wedge compressed in the standard fashion.
- ○ Final fluoroscopic assessment confirms the desired coronal plane correction as well as correct screw placement (**Fig. 10**).

Less commonly, a tibial-sided correction is performed, either to address a primary tibial deformity or along with a distal femoral osteotomy to prevent creating an abnormal joint line obliquity. In these rare circumstances, either a lateral opening or a medial closing wedge technique may be used (**Fig. 11**).

POSTOPERATIVE REGIMEN

- Touch weight bearing for the initial 2 weeks postoperatively then protected weight bearing until 6 weeks
- Hinged knee brace for 6 weeks (unlocked)
- Thrombosis prophylaxis with aspirin
- Immediate initiation of quads activation and knee range-of-motion exercises in brace
- Return to activity 12 weeks postoperatively (low impact) and 24 weeks postoperatively (high impact)

COMPLICATIONS

Besides the general complication profile of bone surgery on the lower extremities, several complications specific to high tibial osteotomy and DFO have been reported in the literature (**Table 2**).[20,23,26,27,33,34]

SUMMARY

Patients with patella instability require thorough clinical assessment to identify and quantify all possible bony and soft tissue contributing factors. Valgus alignment, where pronounced or in the setting of revision surgery, is corrected effectively via osteotomy at the site of deformity. For femoral-sided corrections, MCWDFO is preferred to the stability conferred by the osteotomy design. A low threshold is given to the addition of a soft tissue procedure, most commonly MPFL reconstruction.

CLINICS CARE POINTS

- Particular attention must be paid to the presence of untreated valgus in the setting of revision surgery.
- Consider the need for combining corrective osteotomy with a soft tissue procedure where indicated.
- The presence of a J sign may indicate complex deformity and can be associated with increased risk of isolated MPFL reconstruction failure.
- Beware apparent valgus in long leg standing films. Ensure it has been taken with the femur positioned correctly and that there are not rotational deformities present.
- Be careful not to overcorrect. Correction planning occurs at the joint level but the osteotomy is performed in the metaphysis.
- A medial closing wedge DFO provides a stable osteotomy for early weight bearing with a lower rate of hardware removal.

DISCLOSURE

No disclosure relevant to the current work.

REFERENCES

1. Purushothaman B, Agarwal A, Dawson M. Posttraumatic chronic patellar disloca-tion treated by distal femoral osteotomy and medial patellofemoral ligament reconstruction. Orthopedics 2012;35(11). https://doi.org/10.3928/01477447-20121023-30.
2. Kwon JH, Kim JI, Seo DH, et al. Patellar dislocation with genu valgum treated by DFO. Orthopedics 2013;36(6):840–3.
3. Boden BP, Pearsall AW, Garrett WE, et al. Patellofemoral instability: evaluation and management. J Am Acad Orthop Surg 1997;5(1):47–57. Available at: https://journals.lww.com/jaaos/Fulltext/1997/01000/Patellofemoral_Instability__Ev aluation_and.6.aspx.
4. Swarup I, Elattar O, Rozbruch SR. Patellar instability treated with distal femoral osteotomy. Knee 2017;24(3):608–14.
5. Bullek DD, Scuderi L-GR, Insall JN. Case report management of the chronic irre-ducible patellar dislocation in total knee arthroplasty. J Arthroplasty 1996;11(3): 339–45.
6. Puddu G, Cipolla M, Cerullo G, et al. Which osteotomy for a valgus knee? Int Or-thopaedics 2010;34(2 SPECIAL ISSUE):239–47.
7. Brinkman JM, Freiling D, Lobenhoffer P, et al. Suprakondyläre Femurosteotomien in Kniegelenknähe: Patientenauswahl, Planung, Operationstechniken, Fixations-stabilität und Knochenheilung. Orthopade 2014;43(1):1–10.
8. Joel Finkelstein BA, Gross AE, Davis A. Varus osteotomy of the distal part of the femur a survivorship analysis*. J Bone Joint Surg Am 1996;78(9):1348–52.
9. Nha KW, Ha Y, Oh S, et al. Surgical treatment with closing-wedge distal femoral osteotomy for recurrent patellar dislocation with genu valgum. Am J Sports Med 2018;46(7):1632–40.
10. Wang J-W, Hsu C-C. Distal femoral varus osteotomy for osteoarthritis of the knee. JBJS 2005;87(1):127–33. https://journals.lww.com/jbjsjournal/Fulltext/2005/01000/Distal_Femoral_Varus_Osteotomy_for_Osteoarthritis.18.aspx.
11. Noda M, Saegusa Y, Kashiwagi N, et al. Surgical treatment for permanent dislo-cation of the patella in adults. Orthopedics 2011;34(12). https://doi.org/10.3928/01477447-20111021-27.
12. Chang CB, Shetty GM, Lee JS, et al. A combined closing wedge distal femoral osteotomy and medial reefing procedure for recurrent patellar dislocation with genu valgum. Yonsei Med J 2017;58(4):878–83.
13. Dickschas J, Ferner F, Lutter C, et al. Patellofemoral dysbalance and genua valga: outcome after femoral varisation osteotomies. Arch Orthopaedic Trauma Surg 2018;138(1):19–25.
14. Wilson PL, Black SR, Ellis HB, et al. Distal femoral valgus and recurrent traumatic patellar instability: is an isolated varus producing distal femoral osteotomy a treat-ment option? J Pediatr Orthopaedics 2018;38(3):e162–7.
15. Sabbag OD, Woodmass JM, Wu IT, et al. Medial closing-wedge distal femoral os-teotomy with medial patellofemoral ligament imbrication for genu valgum with lateral patellar instability. Arthrosc Tech 2017;6(6):e2085–91.
16. Kwak JH, Sim JA, Kim NK, et al. Surgical treatment of habitual patella dislocation with genu valgum. Knee Surg Relat Res 2011;23(3):177–9.

17. Imhoff FB, Schnell J, Magaña A, et al. Single cut distal femoral osteotomy for correction of femoral torsion and valgus malformity in patellofemoral malalignment - proof of application of new trigonometrical calculations and 3D-printed cutting guides. BMC Musculoskelet Disord 2018;19(1). https://doi.org/10.1186/s12891-018-2140-5.

18. Hinterwimmer S, Minzlaff P, Saier T, et al. Biplanar supracondylar femoral derotation osteotomy for patellofemoral malalignment: the anterior closed-wedge technique. Knee Surg Sports Traumatol Arthrosc 2014;22(10):2518–21.

19. Robin G, Gozalez-Lomas G. Soft-tissue injuries about the knee. In: Lisa Cannada, editor. Orthopaedc Knowledge Update. American Academy of Orthopaedic Surgeons; 2014.

20. Sheehan FT, Derasari A, Fine KM, et al. Q-angle and J-sign: indicative of maltracking subgroups in patellofemoral pain. Clin Orthopaedics Relat Res 2010; 468(1):266–75.

21. Zhang Z, Zhang H, Song G, et al. A high-grade j sign is more likely to yield higher postoperative patellar laxity and residual maltracking in patients with recurrent patellar dislocation treated with derotational distal femoral osteotomy. The Am J Sports Med 2019;48(1):117–27.

22. Sappey-Marinier E, Sonnery-Cottet B, O'Loughlin P, et al. Clinical outcomes and predictive factors for failure with isolated mpfl reconstruction for recurrent patellar instability: a series of 211 reconstructions with a minimum follow-up of 3 years. Am J Sports Med 2019;47(6):1323–30.

23. Puddu G, Cipolla M, Cerullo G, et al. Osteotomies: the surgical treatment of the valgus knee. Sports Med Arthrosc Rev 2007;15(1):15–22.

24. Cooke TDv, Li J, Scudamore RA. Radiographic assessment of bony contributions to knee deformity. Orthop Clin North Am 1994;25(3). https://doi.org/10.1016/S0030-5898(20)31923-4.

25. SHOJI H, INSALL J. High tibial osteotomy for osteoarthritis of the knee with valgus deformity. JBJS 1973;55(5). Available at: https://journals.lww.com/jbjsjournal/Fulltext/1973/55050/High_Tibial_Osteotomy_for_Osteoarthritis_of_the.5.aspx.

26. Coventry MB. Proximal tibial varus osteotomy for osteoarthritis of the lateral compartment of the knee. J bone Jt Surg Am volume 1987;69(1):32–8. Available at: http://europepmc.org/abstract/MED/3805069.

27. Collins B, Getgood A, Alomar AZ, et al. A case series of lateral opening wedge high tibial osteotomy for valgus malalignment. Knee Surg Sports Traumatol Arthrosc 2013;21(1):152–60.

28. Chambat P, Selmi TAS, Dejour D, et al. Varus tibial osteotomy. Oper Tech Sports Med 2000;8(1):44–7.

29. Saragaglia D, Nemer C, Colle P-E. Computer-assisted double level osteotomy for severe genu varum. Sports Med Arthrosc Rev 2008;16(2). Available at: https://journals.lww.com/sportsmedarthro/Fulltext/2008/06000/Computer_assisted_Double_Level_Osteotomy_for.6.aspx.

30. Babis GC, An K-N, Chao EYS, et al. Double level osteotomy of the knee: a method to retain joint-line obliquity: clinical results. JBJS 2002;84(8). https://journals.lww.com/jbjsjournal/Fulltext/2002/08000/Double_Level_Osteotomy_of_the_Knee__A_Method_to.14.aspx.

31. Paley D. Principles of deformity correction. Springer-Verlag; 2002.

32. Hofmann S, Lobenhoffer P, Staubli A, et al. Osteotomies of the knee joint in patients with monocompartmental arthritis. Orthopade 2009;38(8):755–70.

33. Wylie JD, Jones DL, Hartley MK, et al. Distal femoral osteotomy for the valgus knee: medial closing wedge versus lateral opening wedge: a systematic review. Arthrosc - J Arthroscopic Relat Surg 2016;32(10):2141–7.
34. Chahla J, Mitchell JJ, Liechti DJ, et al. Opening- and closing-wedge distal femoral osteotomy: a systematic review of outcomes for isolated lateral compartment osteoarthritis. Orthopaedic J Sports Med 2016;4(6). https://doi.org/10.1177/2325967116649901.
35. Saithna A, Kundra R, Getgood A, et al. Opening wedge distal femoral varus osteotomy for lateral compartment osteoarthritis in the valgus knee. Knee 2014; 21(1):172–5. https://doi.org/10.1016/j.knee.2013.08.014.
36. Brinkman JM, Hurschler C, Staubli AE, et al. Axial and torsional stability of an improved single-plane and a new bi-plane osteotomy technique for supracondylar femur osteotomies. Knee Surg Sports Traumatol Arthrosc 2011;19(7):1090–8. https://doi.org/10.1007/s00167-010-1349-0.
37. van Heerwaarden R, Najfeld M, Brinkman M, et al. Wedge volume and osteotomy surface depend on surgical technique for distal femoral osteotomy. Knee Surg Sports Traumatol Arthrosc 2013;21(1):206–12. https://doi.org/10.1007/s00167-012-2127-y.
38. Pape D, Dueck K, Haag M, et al. Wedge volume and osteotomy surface depend on surgical technique for high tibial osteotomy. Knee Surg Sports Traumatol Arthrosc 2013;21(1):127–33. https://doi.org/10.1007/s00167-012-1913-x.
39. Imhoff FB, Beitzel K, Zakko P, et al. Derotational osteotomy of the distal femur for the treatment of patellofemoral instability simultaneously leads to the correction of frontal alignment a laboratory cadaveric study. doi:10.1177/2325967118775664
40. Tan SHS, Hui SJ, Doshi C, et al. The outcomes of distal femoral varus osteotomy in patellofemoral instability: a systematic review and meta-analysis. J Knee Surg 2020;33(5):504–12.
41. Dugdale TW, Noyes FR, Styer D. Preoperative planning for high tibial osteotomy. The effect of lateral tibiofemoral separation and tibiofemoral length. Clin orthopaedics Relat Res 1992;274:248–64. http://europepmc.org/abstract/MED/1729010.

Patella Alta

When to Correct and Impact on Other Anatomic Risk Factors for Patellofemoral Instability

Roland M. Biedert, MD

KEYWORDS

- Patella alta • Patellofemoral instability • Trochlear dysplasia
- Rotational abnormalities • Treatment • Osteotomies • Distalization

KEY POINTS

- Patella alta has a decreased patellotrochlear cartilage overlap and represents a predisposing factor for symptomatic patellofemoral instability.
- Patella alta is defined as CDI greater than 1.2, ISI greater than 1.3, and PTI less than 0.125 to 0.28.
- Indications for surgical correction are mostly based on the CDI (>1.2) and the PTI (<0.125–0.28).
- The desired postoperative patellar height is CDI of 1.0 to 1.2, PTI of 0.3 to 0.4, and ISI of 0.95.
- Patella alta has a strong impact on other risk factors for patellofemoral instability and vice versa.

INTRODUCTION

Different morphologic abnormalities, such as patella alta, trochlear dysplasia, rotational abnormalities, excessive tibial tubercle-trochlear groove (TT-TG) distance, patellar tilt, and hypermobility, are predisposing factors for symptomatic patellofemoral (PF) instability.[1–5] They are present alone or in variable combinations and differently affect patellar kinematics.[6] A precise assessment of the pathologic anatomy and modified biomechanics of PF instability is therefore essential for improved understanding of the altered forces acting on the axial, coronal, and sagittal plane and for optimal treatment. Considering this, individually tailored surgical correction may be necessary for successful outcomes in patients with long-term complaints and failed conservative treatment.

Patella alta is described as abnormally high-riding patella in relation to the femur, the TG, or the tibia with decreased bony stability.[7–11] Typically, patella alta has a reduced

---

SportsClinic#1, Wankdorf Center, Papiermühlestrasse 73, CH-3014 Bern, Switzerland
E-mail addresses: biedert@sportsclinicnumber1.ch; r.biedert@bluewin.ch

Clin Sports Med 41 (2022) 65–76
https://doi.org/10.1016/j.csm.2021.07.002

articular area of PF contact with decreased patellotrochlear cartilage overlap.[1,12–14] Sometimes the patella sits even out of the trochlea, especially with quadriceps muscle contracted, and is associated with increased lateral translation.[14] An abnormally high positioned patella may therefore insufficiently engage the proximal TG in extension and early knee flexion. Accordingly, patella alta is one of the potential risk factors for PF instability.[5,10,15–17] In addition, it is also observed in patients with PF pain, chondromalacia, Sinding-Larsen-Johansson disease, Osgood-Schlatter disease, patellar tendinopathy, and osteoarthritis representing also an important predisposing factor for patellar malalignment and PF-related complaints.[1,6,7,13,16,18,19] In contrast, patella alta may also be a normal variant of individual knee anatomy and is well tolerated without additional instability factors.[5]

In the normal knee, the patella enhances functionally the lever arm of the extensor mechanism.[20] During the range of motion, high loads transfer to the articular side of the patella. The contact point changes between patella and trochlea during flexion-extension movements and the joint reaction forces (JRF) change because of altered force vectors in the lever system.[20] The thick articular cartilage of the patella dissipates large JRF during contractions of the quadriceps muscle.

In patients with patella alta, joint kinematics and cartilage contact position are altered caused by a modified lever arm between quadriceps and patellar tendon.[21] Patella alta is correlated with a larger quadriceps and smaller patellar tendon moment arm with a greater transmission force from quadriceps to patellar tendon.[16,22] A posteriorly directed force on the patella is generated by the altered pulls of the quadriceps tendon and the patellar tendon and supraphysiologic lateral force vectors can result.[20] The altered position of the patella may lead to elevated PF joint contact stress because of smaller contact area and increased JRF in deeper knee flexion resulting in cartilage damage, PF pain, or complaints.[14,23]

MEASUREMENT METHODS

Overall, four different types of measurement methods are used to assess patella alta: (1) lateral radiographs with corresponding ratios, (2) radiograph ratios measured on MRI, (3) patellotrochlear index (PTI) on sagittal MRI, and (4) patellar tendon length measurement.[1] The cutoff values for patella alta according to the specific measurement method are summarized in **Box 1**.[1,10,12,24] However, there is still no generally accepted consensus for any measurement method or cutoff value for patella alta.

Box 1
Measurement methods for patella alta with cutoff values

Radiograph measurements
- Caton-Deschamps index >1.2
- Insall-Salvati index >1.3
- Blackburne-Peel index >1.0

Radiograph ratios on sagittal MRI sequences
- Caton-Deschamps index >1.2
- Insall-Salvati index >1.3

Sagittal MRI (central cut)
- PTI <0.125–0.28

Sagittal MRI (longest patella axis)
- Patellar tendon length (Insall-Salvati index) >52 mm

The radiograph measurement indices mark the position of the patella relative to the tibia.[1,12] The variable bony morphologies of patella (distal patella nose, different articulating surface, fragmentation distal patellar bone), femoral trochlea (facet in length and height), proximal tibia (TT deformities, fragmentation, hypertrophy), and slope are confounding factors that may affect measurement.[1] Specific variations in PF morphology (eg, small articular surface, short trochlea) are not represented by these indices. Therefore, correct measurement for patella alta should preferably relate the position of the patella to the femur rather than the tibia.[25]

In addition, the real articular PF relationship is not sufficiently assessed because articular cartilage is not visible on radiographs (**Fig. 1**).[1,12,19] The cartilaginous overlap between trochlea and patella represents the most relevant factor for patella alta and should be measured using MRI.[5,10,12,19] Therefore, the use of the PTI is recommended for precise assessment (**Fig. 2**). The PTI traces preoperative and postoperative values, which makes these measurements valuable.

Using radiograph measurements only, the Caton-Deschamps index (CDI) is superior to the Insall-Salvati index (ISI), especially when considering surgical correction with distalization of the TT.[1]

The CDI assesses the height of the patella relative to the tibial plateau and is therefore the most useful measuring method on radiographs for patellar height before and

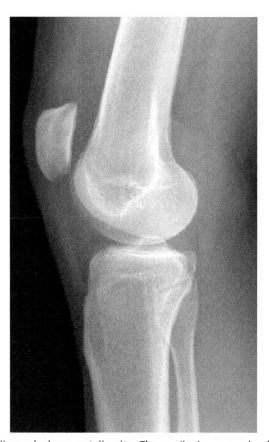

Fig. 1. Lateral radiograph shows patella alta. The cartilaginous overlap between trochlea and patella is not visible.

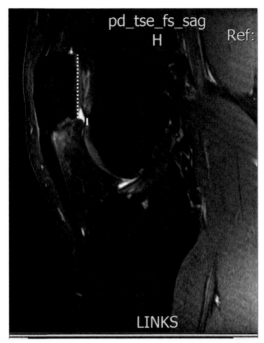

Fig. 2. Patellotrochlear index measured on sagittal MRI (central cut) shows the missing true articular patella (*dotted line*), and trochlea (*solid line*) overlap in patella alta with impingement of the Hoffa fat pad.

after distalization of the TT.[1] The ISI does not change after distalization of the TT and therefore cannot be recommended.[1]

CORRECTION OF PATELLA ALTA

Treatment of patella alta is conservative at the beginning. The focus is on improved functional stability, coordination, and strength. The patella is externally stabilized using kinesiotape or soft brace to reduce symptoms during practice.

Surgical correction of patella alta is indicated in patients with a long history of ongoing symptoms, unsuccessful conservative treatment over a long period, functional disability, clinical examination findings, and documentation by imaging. The ideal surgical procedure to address patella alta should restore biomechanics of the extensor mechanism of the knee and increase PF stability.[23] In addition, PF joint contact stress and JRF should normalize. The appropriate procedure depends on the patient's anatomy, pathomorphology, and age. Various combinations are used to address all causes of instability or complaints.

Indications by Measurements

The different surgical procedures to correct patella alta are primarily based on the CDI and the PTI,[1,10] more rarely on the ISI (**Table 1**).

Surgical Procedures

Two types of surgical procedures are used to correct patella alta: TT osteotomies and soft tissue methods.

Table 1
Indications to treat patella alta[1,12]

Measurement	Ratio	Reference
CDI	>1.2	3,26
	>1.3	27
	>1.4	28–30
ISI	>1.3	26
PTI	<0.125–0.28	1,12
	<0.18	10
Radiograph ratios on sagittal MRI sequences		
CDI	>1.2	
ISI	>1.3	24

Transfers of the tibial tubercle

TT distalization is an effective procedure of normalizing patellar height to correct the patellar index in patella alta.[1,18,27,31,32] TT distalization is indicated in patients with recurrent patellar dislocations, PF pain, Hoffa impingement, and cartilage lesions because of patella alta and facilitates the engagement with the TG at low flexion angles.[1,3,8] It is performed as a single procedure or in combination with other stabilizing interventions. Additional medialization or anteromedialization may be indicated in cases with increased TT-TG distance (>20 mm), cartilage lesions, or osteoarthritis. TT osteotomy is performed in two planes: three-dimensional or V-shaped.[13]

The patellar height, TT-TG distance, and lateral patellar subluxation improve after surgery depending on the amount of correction. Posteriorization must be strictly prevented in order not to increase PF contact forces. Direction and degree of TT transfer must be individually adapted preoperatively according to patient parameters and focus on the goal of the procedure.[33] The amount of the desired distalization is calculated to result in a postoperative CDI of 1.0 to 1.2, and PTI of 0.3 to 0.4 (**Table 2, Fig. 3**).[1,20]

The risk of complications following TT osteotomies, such as nonunion, tibial fractures, overcorrection, posteriorization, skin necrosis, infection, and hardware complications/irritation, is related to the technique used and is between 3.3% and 10.7%.[35]

TT distalization and additional patellar tendon tenodesis attached to its original insertion results in normalization of patellar tendon length and a stable PF joint in patients with patella alta.[34] Comparing these surgical procedures, cartilage stress seems lower using distalization as opposed to distalization and tenodesis.

Soft tissue methods

Patellar tendon imbrication is an effective procedure to correct patella alta in the skeletally immature patient suffering from lateral patellar instability. Soft tissue methods are recommended because bony procedures injure the proximal tibial physis and

Table 2
Desired postoperative patellar height[1,12]

Measurement	Ratio	Reference
Caton-Deschamps index (on radiographs)	1.0–1.1–1.2	20,27,29
Patellotrochlear index (MRI)	0.3–0.4	1
Insall-Salvati index	0.95	18,34

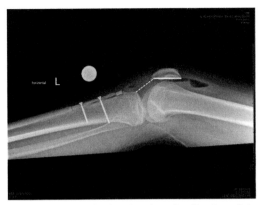

Fig. 3. Lateral radiograph shows patellar height after distalization of the tibial tubercle. The distally removed bone block is inserted proximally to stabilize the TT osteotomy. The CDI is 1.0.

may lead to its premature closure.[36] On average, this technique allows 1 cm of patellar tendon shortening.

Distal advancement of the patella can also be achieved by complete mobilization of the patellar tendon and fixed with sutures through the cartilaginous TT. This technique offers a satisfactory treatment of the immature patient presenting with habitual patellar dislocation associated with patella alta.[37]

IMPACT ON OTHER ANATOMIC RISK FACTORS

Patella alta may also be present in combination with other risk factors for patellar instability. The variable combinations of deformities affect patellar kinematics in different ways.[6] Therefore, the impacts on the specific risk factors for patellar instability must be assessed to determine the best treatment.

Anatomic Risk Factors

Trochlear dysplasia

Trochlear dysplasia is an abnormality of shape and depth of the TG with variable length of the articular zone.[3,5,17,37] Different forms of trochlear dysplasia are described, such as decreased depth, decreased inclination of the lateral facet, flat trochlea, trochlear bump (anterior translation of the trochlear floor), and hypoplasia of the medial trochlea. These forms of trochlear variations are located proximally and cause decreased bony stability in the TG. The patella is insufficiently guided at the entrance into the trochlea in extension and at the beginning of knee flexion and lateral instability with increased lateral tilt may occur.

Patella alta and trochlear dysplasia (type C and D) in combination represent a severe pathomorphology with two different instability factors resulting in reduced lateral mechanical joint stability (**Fig. 4** A and B).[38] TT distalization alone would only correct patellar height, but not significantly improve joint stability because of the dysplastic groove, which fails to provide lateral constraint. The engagement of the patella into the dysplastic sulcus (flat or even prominent anterior bump) would still be prevented in extension and early knee flexion. Therefore, deepening trochleoplasty to establish a concave surface of correct depth, length, and sulcus orientation on the proximal trochlea may be necessary at the same time to improve patellar

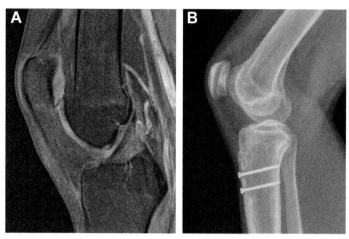

Fig. 4. (*A*) Sagittal MRI showing patella alta (PTI 0.14) and trochlear dysplasia type D with prominent supratrochlear spur. (*B*) Postoperative lateral radiograph after distalization of the tibial tubercle showing normal patellar height and after deepening trochleoplasty (same patient as Fig. 4A).

stability. When performing deepening trochleoplasty it is also possible to reduce the TT-TG distance.[4] In some cases, only mild deepening may be necessary at the proximal entrance of the trochlea. With this, the contact area increases and the PF contact pressure decreases.

Short lateral trochlear facet
A too short proximal-lateral extension of the articular trochlear facet represents another type of trochlear dysplasia in the coronal plane.[37] The patella is well centered in the trochlea under relaxed conditions. Muscular contraction of the extensor mechanism leads to proximalization and lateralization of the patella resulting in dynamic lateral subluxation. The lateral subluxation of the patella is caused by the missing osteochondral opposing force of the too short lateral trochlear facet (**Fig. 5**). With increasing knee flexion, the patella enters into the more distal and normal part of the TG and becomes therefore more stable. But in combination with patella alta, the lateral patellar instability is significantly increased because of the missing lateral facet contact and already present under relaxed conditions.

TT distalization alone would result in normal patellar height and improved joint stability, but only under relaxed conditions. Therefore, proximal-lateral trochlear lengthening osteotomy is recommended at the same time to improve also the dynamic stability in this combination.[4,37]

Torsional abnormalities
Torsional abnormalities influence the PF kinematics and cause altered vectors and forces acting on the PF joint.[39,40] Increased femoral antetorsion represents a significant etiologic factor causing lateral patellar instability.[39–42] The knee joint is pointed internally and the pull on the quadriceps is lateral.[40] This increases the lateral trochlea facet compression and may cause lateral patellar instability.

In combination with patella alta, the counterforce against lateral patellar instability is decreased or absent because of the missing lateral facet contact and the instability becomes more significant.

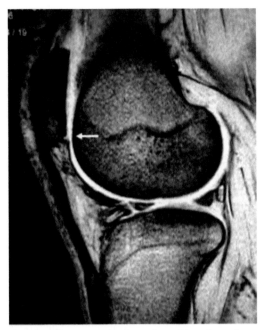

Fig. 5. Sagittal MRI showing short anterior lateral trochlear facet (*arrow*) with no patello-trochlear cartilage overlap and patella alta. The PTI is 0, the CDI is 1.3, and the lateral condyle index is 66%.[37]

Treating patella alta by distalization would increase patella stability, but only until the failure rate of the medial PF ligament (MPFL) is reached. Combined insufficiency of the MPFL and increased femoral antetorsion (>25°–30°) may result in symptomatic patellar instability by itself. In combination with patella alta, the instability and secondary effects become worse and combined surgical correction consisting of TT distalization and femoral derotation osteotomy may be considered.

Excessive tibial tubercle-trochlear groove distance
A lateral insertion of the patellar tendon on the tibia is considered as one of the main factors of patellar instability. This is quantified as the medial-lateral TT-TG distance. A threshold of 20 mm or more signifies an abnormal value.[4,6,17,20] In combination with patella alta, the reduced engagement of the patella with the TG and the increased TT-TG distance result in elevated lateral shift, tilt, and instability of the patella. This typically increases with knee extension because of the tibial external rotation of the screw-home mechanism.[43] In addition, the interaction of TT lateralization combined with patella alta significantly increases the amount of anisometry seen in the reconstructed MPFL, with almost 5 mm of mean maximal length change demonstrated with the combination of TT-TG of 25 mm and CDI of 1.4.[44] Distalization combined with TT medialization restores the engagement of the patella with the TG and reduces patellar lateral shift. With this, the risk of patellar instability is decreased especially near full extension. Overcorrection to medial and/or posteriorization of the TT must be strictly avoided. The use of the tubercle-sulcus angle assessed in 90° of knee flexion may be helpful.

Valgus knee
Excessive valgus knee alignment determines increased lateral patellar displacement with higher risk of dynamic patellar instability, especially close to extension and during

quadriceps contraction. This negative effect is exacerbated by the presence of a patella alta at the same time. In this condition, the laterally pulled patella lays completely above the trochlea without osseous support preventing lateral subluxation or dislocation. This results in a multifactorial lateral patellar instability.

Distalization of patella alta improves the bony support in the TG and decreases patellar instability despite the laterally oriented force vectors given by the valgus knee. In cases with excessive genu valgum, femoral varisation (varus producing) osteotomy may be indicated at the same time.[45]

Medial patellofemoral ligament insufficiency

The MPFL is the most important static soft tissue provider of passive lateral stability for the patella (50%–60%).[46,47] The MPFL acts as a checkrein during the first 30° of knee flexion before the patella engaging the TG.[48] In patients with patella alta, the MPFL may be insufficient because of the lateral patellar instability. Patella alta significantly alters MPFL anatomometry.[44] A reconstruction performed at Schoettle point (as in patients with normal patellar height) would therefore fail to produce a truly anatomometric MPFL. Proximalization of the femoral attachment site of MPFL reconstruction may be necessary.[44] TT distalization alone should not be expected to completely correct the instability and MPFL reconstruction or double-breasting reefing must be added. Poor graft positioning should be strictly avoided because misplaced femoral tunnels dramatically increase maximum contact pressures within the PF joint.[48]

However, persistent patella alta after MPFL reconstruction results in decreased lateral restraining forces, PF contact area, and increased maximum PF contact pressures, which could explain clinical failures of isolated MPFL reconstruction in the setting of patella alta.[48] This underlines the importance of TT distalization in patients with patellar instability and the combination of patella alta and MPFL insufficiency.

Hypermobility

In patients with patella alta and hypermobility, the elasticity of the ligaments allows for increased lateral displacement of the patella because the bony stability of the TG is missing at the same time. This phenomenon is increased with quadriceps contraction. Patella hypermobility occurs more frequently in patients with patellar dislocation compared with the general population.[14,49] This indicates that soft tissue plays an important role in stabilization of the patella, especially at full knee extension when the patella is superior to the bony restraint of the TG.[46]

Performing distalization of the patella, the patella enters into the trochlea and becomes more stable. Nevertheless, it is recommended to shorten and double-breast the lax ligaments on the medial side at the same time.

CLINICS CARE POINTS

- Different morphologic abnormalities are predisposing factors for patellofemoral instability.
- Patella alta with insufficient engagement of the patella in the trochlea is a most important one.
- Correct imaging assessment of all patella instability factors is mandatory to determine optimal treatment.
- All morphologic, biomechanic, and functional factors must be addressed during surgical correction for successful outcome.

DISCLOSURE

The author has nothing to disclose.

INSTITUTIONAL REVIEW BOARD STATEMENT

This study did not require ethical approval.

REFERENCES

1. Biedert RM, Tscholl PM. Patella alta: a comprehensive review of current knowledge. Am J Orthop 2017;46:290–300.
2. Van Huyssteen AL, Hendrix MRG, Barnet AJ, et al. Cartilage-bone mismatch in the dysplastic trochlea. J Bone Joint Surg Br 2006;88:688–91.
3. Dejour D, Le Coultre B. Osteotomies in patello-femoral instabilities. Sports Med Arthrosc Rev 2007;15:39–46.
4. McNamara I, Bua N, Smith TO, et al. Deepening trochleoplasty with a thick osteochondral flap for patellar instability: clinical and functional outcomes at a mean 6-year follow-up. Am J Sports Med 2015;43:2706–13.
5. Askenberger M, Janarv PM, Finnbogason T, et al. Morphology and anatomic patellar instability risk factors in first-time traumatic lateral patellar dislocations. Am J Sports Med 2017;45:50–8.
6. Steensen RN, Bentley JC, Trinh TQ, et al. The prevalence and combined prevalences of anatomic factors associated with recurrent patellar dislocation: a magnetic resonance imaging study. Am J Sports Med 2015;43:921–7.
7. Munch JL, Sullivan JP, Nguyen JT, et al. Patellar articular overlap on MRI is a simple alternative to conventional measurements of patellar height. Orthop J Sports Med 2016;4:1–6.
8. Elias JJ, Soehnlen NT, Guseila LM, et al. Dynamic tracking influenced by anatomy in patellar instability. Knee 2016;23:450–5.
9. Fabricant PD, Ladenhauf HN, Salvati EA, et al. Medial patellofemoral ligament (MPFL) reconstruction improves radiographic measures of patella alta in children. Knee 2014;21:1180–4.
10. Ali SA, Helmer R, Terk MR. Patella alta: lack of correlation between patellotrochlear cartilage congruence and commonly used patellar height ratios. AJR Am J Roentgenol 2009;193:1361–6.
11. Verhulst F, van Sambeeck J, Olthuis G, et al. Patellar height measurements: Insall-Salvati ratio is most reliable method. Knee Surg Sports Traumatol Arthrosc 2020; 28:869–75.
12. Biedert RM, Albrecht S. The patellotrochlear index: a new index for assessing patellar height. Knee Surg Sports Traumatol Arthrosc 2006;14:707–12.
13. Otsuki S, Nakajima M, Fujiwara K, et al. Influence of age on clinical outcomes of three-dimensional transfer of the tibial tuberosity for patellar instability with patella alta. Knee Surg Sports Traumatol Arthrosc 2017;25:2392–6.
14. Wheatley G, Rainbow J, Clouthier A. Patellofemoral mechanics: a review of pathomechanics and research approaches. Curr Rev Musculoskelet Med 2020;13: 326–37.
15. Mayer C, Magnussen RA, Servien E, et al. Patellar tendon tenodesis in association with tibial tubercle distalization for the treatment of episodic patellar dislocation with patella alta. Am J Sports Med 2012;40:346–51.

16. Ward SR, Terk MR, Powers CM. Patella alta: association with patellofemoral alignment and changes in contact area during weight-bearing. J Bone Joint Surg Am 2007;89:1749–55.

17. Dejour H, Walch G, Nove-Josserand L, et al. Factors of patellar instability: an anatomic radiographic study. Knee Surg Sports Traumatol Arthrosc 1994;2: 19–26.

18. Yin L, Liao TC, Yang L, et al. Does patella tendon tenodesis improve tibial tubercle distalization in treating patella alta? A computational study. Clin Orthop Rel Res 2016;474:2451–61.

19. Barnett AJ, Prentice M, Mandalia V, et al. Patellar height measurement in trochlear dysplasia. Knee Surg Sports Traumatol Arthrosc 2009;17:1412–5.

20. Middleton KK, Gruber S, Shubin S, et al. Why and where to move the tibial tubercle. Sports Med Arthrosc Rev 2019;27:154–60.

21. Dan M, Parr W, Broe D, et al. Biomechanics of the knee extensor mechanism and its relationship to patella tendinopathy: a review. J Orthop Res 2018;36:3105–12.

22. Ward SR, Powers CM. The influence of patella alta on patellofemoral joint stress during normal and fast walking. Clin Biomech 2004;19:1040–7.

23. Seidl A, Baldini T, Krughoff K, et al. Biomechanical assessment of patellar advancement procedures for patella alta. Orthopedics 2016;39:492–7.

24. Miller TT, Staron RB, Feldman F. Patellar height on sagittal MR imaging of the knee. AJR Am J Roentgenol 1996;167:339–41.

25. Rosa SB, Bahho Z, Doma K, et al. The quadriceps active ratio: a dynamic MRI-based assessment of patellar height. Eur J Orthop Surg Traumatol 2018;28: 1165–74.

26. Feller JA. Distal realignment (tibial tuberosity transfer). Sports Med Arthrosc Rev 2012;20:152–61.

27. Dietrich TJ, Fucentese SF, Pfirrmann CW. Imaging of individual anatomical risk factors for patellar instability. Semin Musculoskelet Radiol 2016;20:65–73.

28. Dean CS, Chahla J, Serra Cruz R, et al. Patellofemoral joint reconstruction for patellar instability: medial patellofemoral ligament reconstruction, trochleoplasty, and tibial tubercle osteotomy. Arthrosc Tech 2016;5:169–75.

29. Frosch KH, Schmeling A. A new classification system of patellar instability and patellar maltracking. Arch Orthop Trauma Surg 2016;136:485–97.

30. Weber AE, Nathani A, Dines JS, et al. An algorithmic approach to the management of recurrent lateral patellar dislocation. J Bone Joint Surg Am 2016;98: 417–27.

31. Park MS, Chung CY, Lee KM, et al. Which is the best method to determine the patellar height in children and adolescents? Clin Orthop Relat Res 2010;468: 1344–51.

32. Edama M, Kageyama I, Nakamura M, et al. Anatomical study of the inferior patellar pole and patellar tendon. Scand J Med Sci Sports 2017;27:1681–7.

33. Grimm NL, Lazarides AL, Amendola A. Tibial tubercle osteotomies: a review of a treatment for recurrent patellar instability. Curr Rev Musculoskelet Med 2018;11: 266–71.

34. Neyret Ph, Robinson N, Le Coultre B, et al. Patellar tendon length: the factor in patellar instability? Knee 2002;9:3–6.

35. Rood A, van Sambeeck J, Koëter S, et al. A detaching, V-shaped tibial tubercle osteotomy is a safe procedure with a low complication rate. Arch Orthop Trauma Surg 2020;140:1867–72.

36. Patel R, Gombosh M, Polster J, et al. Patellar tendon imbrication is a safe and efficacious technique to shorten the patellar tendon in patients with patella alta. Orthop J Sports Med 2020;27(8). 2325967120959318.
37. Biedert RM, Netzer P, Gal I, et al. The lateral condyle index: a new index for assessing the length of the lateral articular trochlea as predisposing factor for patellar instability. Int Orthop 2011;35:1327–31.
38. Van Haver A, De Roo K, De Beule M, et al. The effect of trochlear dysplasia on patellofemoral biomechanics: a cadaveric study with simulated trochlear deformities. Am J Sports Med 2015;43:1354–61.
39. Teitge RA. Osteotomy in the treatment of patellofemoral instability. Tech Knee Surg 2006;5:2–18.
40. Teitge RA. The role of limb rotational osteotomy in the treatment of patellofemoral dysfunction. In: Zaffagnini S, Dejour D, Arendt EA, editors. Patellofemoral pain, instability, and arthritis. England: Springer; 2010. p. 237–44.
41. Yoshioka Y, Cooke TDV. Femoral anteversion: assessment based on function axes. J Orthop Res 1987;5:86–91.
42. Imhoff FB, Cotic M, Liska F, et al. Derotational osteotomy at the distal femur is effective to treat patients with patellar instability. Knee Surg Sports Traumatol Arthosc 2019;27:652–8.
43. Elias JJ, Carrino JA, Saranathan A, et al. Variations in kinematics and function following patellar stabilization including tibial tuberosity realignment. Knee Surg Sports Traumatol Arthrosc 2014;22:2350–6.
44. Belkin NS, Meyers KN, Redler LH, et al. Medial patellofemoral ligament isometry in the setting of patella alta. Arthroscopy 2020;36(12):3031–6.
45. Dickschas J, Ferner F, Lutter C, et al. Patellofemoral dysbalance and genua valga: outcome after femoral varisation osteotomies. Arch Orthop Trauma Surg 2018;138:19–25.
46. Amis AA. Current concepts on anatomy and biomechanics of patellar stability. Sports Med Arthrosc Rev 2007;15:48–56.
47. Tanaka MJ, Voss A, Fulkerson JP. The anatomic midpoint of the attachment of the medial patellofemoral complex. J Bone Joint Surg Am 2016;98:1199–205.
48. Watson NA, Duchman KR, Grosland NM, et al. Finite element analysis of patella alta: a patellofemoral instability model. Iowa Orthop J 2017;37:101–8.
49. Nomura E, Inoue M, Kobayashi S. Generalized joint laxity and contralateral patellar hypermobility in unilateral recurrent patellar dislocators. Arthroscopy 2006;22:861–5.

Trochlear Dysplasia
When and How to Correct

Edoardo Giovannetti de Sanctis, MD*, Guillaume Mesnard, MD,
David H. Dejour, MD

KEYWORDS

- Trochlear • Dysplasia • Trochleoplasty • Sulcus • Deepening • Patellar dislocation

KEY POINTS

- When? Only patients with high-grade trochlear dysplasia types B and D, in which the prominence of the trochlea (supratrochlear spur) is over 5 mm, recurrent patellar dislocation, and maltracking.
- How? Sulcus deepening trochleoplasty: modifies the trochlear shape with a central groove and oblique medial and lateral facets; decreases the patellofemoral joint reaction force by reducing the trochlear prominence (spur); and reduces the tibial tubercle and the trochlear groove value by a proximal realignment.
- Pros: This procedure is highly effective in restoring patellofemoral stability and satisfying the patients.
- Cons: The patients must be aware of the risk of continuing residual pain and range-of-motion limitation and that the development of patellofemoral osteoarthritis is not predictable.

WHEN
From Normal to Dysplastic Trochlear Anatomy

The basis of the anatomy describes the femoral trochlea as the cartilaginous anterior part of the distal femur articulating with the patella. It is composed of 2 facets divided by a longitudinal groove, the trochlear sulcus extending distally to the notch. The lateral facet is both larger and more protuberant anteriorly than the medial facet in the coronal and sagittal plane.

The condylotrochlear grooves are the trochlea's distal margins, dividing each facet with the corresponding femoral condyle.

The patella lies on the anterior femoral cortex in full extension and engages the trochlea in early flexion. During flexion, the obliquity of the opposed articulating surfaces in the axial plane and the progressive external rotation of femur produce vector,

Lyon-Ortho-Clinic, Clinique de la Sauvegarde, Ramsay Santé, 8, Avenue Ben Gourion, Lyon 69009, France
* Corresponding author. Lyon Ortho Clinic, 29 Avenue des Sources, Lyon 69009, France.
E-mail address: edoardo.giovannettids@gmail.com

Clin Sports Med 41 (2022) 77–88
https://doi.org/10.1016/j.csm.2021.09.001
0278-5919/22/© 2021 Elsevier Inc. All rights reserved.

directing the patella medially toward the trochlear groove. Furthermore, a posteriorly directed force produced by the quadriceps pushes the patella against the trochlea.

Patellofemoral Instability and Trochlear Dysplasia

Patellar instability can present in 3 different forms: simple traumatic lateral patellar dislocation, recurrent patellar instability, and permanent dislocations. This pathologic condition's risk factors include the following in order of importance: trochlear dysplasia, patella alta, and an excessive distance between the tibial tubercle and the trochlear groove (TT-TG). Other causes of patellar instability to consider include the following: genu valgum, femoral head version, vastus medialis atrophy, and patellar dysplasia.[1]

The trochlear shape, and therefore an incongruency between trochlear and patellar surfaces, has a high influence on patellar tilt, subluxation, and lateral displacement. Trochlear dysplasia refers to a genetic pathologic alteration of the shape of the trochlea, becoming shallow, flat, or convex. Furthermore, a bump in the superolateral aspect is common. The higher the degree of trochlear dysplasia, the higher the risk of instability.

Radiographic Evaluation

Standard radiographic views, such as true sagittal view, skyline view at 30° of flexion, and anteroposterior view, must be evaluated for a correct sulcus deepening trochleoplasty surgical indication. The lateral view must be performed superimposing the 2 posterior femoral condyles in a monopodal weight-bearing position with 20° of flexion. This projection shows from anterior to posterior the contour of the facets and the line representing the trochlear sulcus.[2,3] The lateral condyle, and therefore the lateral facet, might be recognized, having a more visible condylotrochlear groove and a greater radiopacity. The line representing the trochlear sulcus continues with the Blumensaat line, which is the line drawn along the roof of the intercondylar notch.

On the sagittal view, the trochlear dysplasia is defined by the 3 following pillars: the crossing sign, the supratrochlear spur, and the double-contour sign. The crossing sign is defined as the point where the trochlear sulcus radiographic line touches the projection of the anterior femoral condyles. It represents macroscopically the exact position where the sulcus and anterior femoral condyle have the same height, meaning that part of the groove has become flat. The supratrochlear spur and double contour sign represent, respectively, a protuberance (bump or prominence) on the superolateral part of the trochlea and the medial hypoplastic facet, seen as a double line at the anterior aspect of the condyles.

Axial views obtained with the knee flexed 30° might be used to evaluate the shape of the trochlea, measure the sulcus angle, and evaluate the patella dysplasia classified according to Wiberg.[4] From the deepest point of the groove, 2 lines are drawn, toward the most superior point of each condyle. The mean normal sulcus angle value defined by Merchant is 145° ± 6°. In trochlear dysplasia, the sulcus angle is increased or unmeasurable.

The trochlear dysplasia is classified into 4 types using 3 signs.[5,6] The Dejour's classification could be correctly done only if the sagittal radiographic data are cross-checked with the slice image data[1] (**Fig. 1**).

Type A: Crossing sign (radiographs), shallower trochlea (slice images).

Type B: Crossing sign and supratrochlear spur (radiographs), flat or convex trochlea (slice images) (**Fig. 2**).

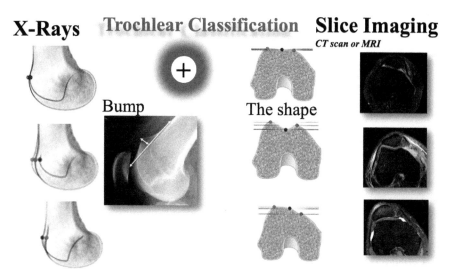

Fig. 1. Dejour's classification needs a combination of radiographs to determine the crossing sign, the supratrochlear spur and the double contour, and slice imaging to determine the shape of the trochlea.

Type C: Crossing sign and double-contour sign (radiographs), convex lateral facet, and hypoplastic medial facet (slice images).

Type D: Crossing sign, supratrochlear spur, and double-contour sign (radiographs), hypoplastic medial facet proximally short and almost absent with a vertical connection to a prominent and convex lateral facet defining the so-called cliff pattern (slice images) (**Fig. 3**).

Slice imaging, such as a computed tomographic (CT) scan or MRI, shows perfectly the global shape of the trochlea: shallow, flat, or convex. Both are able to quantify the axial malalignment (TT-TG) and the patellar tilt. CT scan is better to quantify lower-limb torsion on both sides. The use of arthro-CT quantifies cartilage lesions, especially those on the central patella, with concordance with arthroscopy and arthrotomy in 97.1% of cases, and can reveal any loose bodies.[7] MRI has the advantage of better assessing any softening and/or damage to the cartilage.[8] Using MRI to evaluate the cartilaginous shape of the trochlear groove might be useful, as often the shape of the cartilage lining does not follow exactly the underlying bony anatomy.[9]

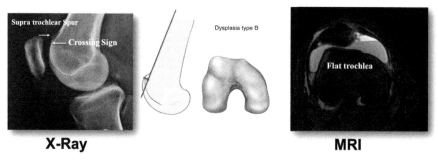

Fig. 2. Type B trochlear dysplasia.

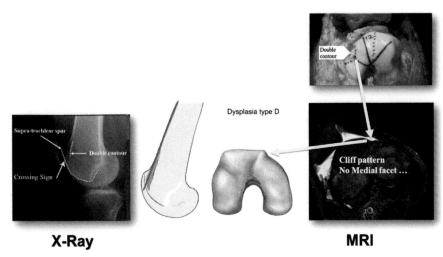

X-Ray   **MRI**

Fig. 3. Type D trochlear dysplasia.

Clinical Evaluation

Anterior knee pain, subjective feeling of an unstable knee, and locking or catching are among the most frequent clinical symptoms in patients with trochlear dysplasia. During static inspection and palpation, the physician should figure out whether the patella is centered within the groove or if it is permanently subluxated/dislocated. Describing all the signs and tests used during clinical evaluation of the patellofemoral joint go beyond the purpose of this article. Only 4 of those are described, which are relevant for the surgical indications and associate procedures: the J-sign, abnormal patellar maltracking, apprehension, and patella tilt test.

The J-sign is evident from extension to early flexion (or vice versa) in a maltracking patella. A laterally subluxated patella suddenly shifts medially, engaging the trochlear groove with the quadriceps contracted. The J-sign during the physical examination is suggestive of patellar maltracking and potential instability and a functional patella alta.

The abnormal patellar maltracking is only seen in high-grade trochlear dysplasia. The patella could dislocate or reduce when the patient does active or passive flexion-extension. If there is a dislocation in extension, the extensor mechanism has no retraction; if there is a dislocation in flexion, the extensor mechanism is too short distally (patella infera) or proximally (quadriceps contraction).

The apprehension test is a physical finding in which forced lateral displacement of the patella produces anxiety and resistance in patients with a history of lateral patellar instability.

The patellar tilt test assesses the amount of patellar tilt that can be elicited by an examiner, giving an idea of the tightness of the retinaculum on each side of the patella. A negative medial tilt test quantifies lateral retinaculum tightening; in high-grade trochlear dysplasia, it is a regular feature, and it means that the lateral retinaculum must be cut or lengthened.

Treatment Algorithm

Sulcus deepening trochleoplasty indications are precise, that is, recurrent patellar dislocations with both high-grade trochlear dysplasia and patellar maltracking. The contraindications are established patello-femoral osteoarthritis, open growth plates, and a painful knee with no dislocations.

Types B and D fit the best with sulcus deepening trochleoplasty, because of the anterolateral prominence (supratrochlear spur). A cutoff of 5 mm for the height of the prominence has been proposed, as an indication for trochleoplasty in major trochlear dysplasia.[10]

In each patient with trochlear dysplasia, the associated abnormalities must be evaluated and surgically corrected when indicated ("menu à la carte"): for example, distalizing and/or medializing the TT according to sagittal and axial patellar alignment. This will improve the rate of success of this procedure.[11,12]

The medial patellofemoral ligament (MPFL) reconstruction is systematically added to the sulcus, deepening trochleoplasty, in order to treat the consequence of the ligament rupture occurred during the first dislocation episode.

HOW
Sulcus Deepening Trochleoplasty

This procedure was first described by Polar in 1890, but since then it has undergone changes. It was modified first by Masse[13] in 1978 and afterward by Dejour and colleagues[14] in 1987. Then, Dejour improved it in 2010.[5] The procedure's main aim is to decrease the trochlear prominence while creating a new groove with a normal depth and orientation.

This procedure is generally performed under both sedation and regional anesthesia. The patient is placed in a supine position with a thigh tourniquet. The operating table has 2 supports (proximal and distal) helping to keep the knee flexed. The entire lower limb, distal to the tourniquet, is prepared and draped.

A straight midline skin incision from the superior patellar pole to the tibiofemoral joint line is performed with the knee flexed 90°. Thereafter, the knee is extended, and an anteromedial approach is carried out in order to simplify trochlear exposure and MPFL reconstruction. If TT transposition must be performed, a double incision might be done in order to limit scar size. The patella and trochlea are then exposed without patellar eversion. The cartilage of both is assessed and classified according to the International Cartilage Repair Society.[15]

An incision along the femorotrochlear osteochondral junction is performed in order to reflect the synovium and periosteum from the cortex, while using an elevator. This is performed to make the anterior femoral cortex visible and determine the amount of deepening to be undertaken. The anterior cortex of the femoral shaft will be the landmark to be followed to make the future trochlea flush with it.

With the anterior distal femur fully exposed, the native (dashed line) trochlear groove is marked with a sterile pen. Two additional divergent lines (dashed lines), representing the lateral and medial facet limits, are drawn, from the notch going laterally, through the condylotrochlear grooves (sulcus terminalis). Those 2 lines must be out of the tibiofemoral articulation.

The planned (continuous line) trochlear groove is marked in a more lateral position according to the preoperative TT-TG value and the anatomic femoral axis.

To access the undersurface of the trochlea, a strip of femoral cortical bone is removed with an osteotome all along the trochlear proximal edge. The strip thickness is equal to the height of the trochlear prominence measured from the anterior femoral cortex (**Fig. 4**). The trochlear undersurface cancellous bone is thus exposed. Subsequently, part of the cancellous bone must be removed from the undersurface of the trochlea.

Using an offset guide-equipped drill, different tunnels are made through the subtrochlear cancellous bone, from proximal to distal (top of the notch) and parallel to the anterior cortex.

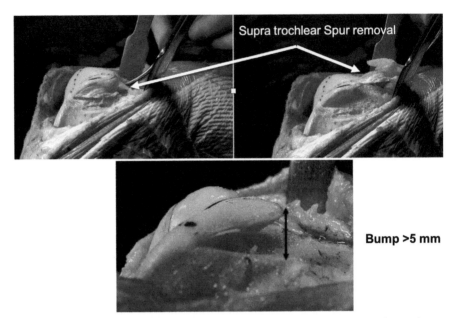

Fig. 4. Supratrochlear spur removal. The new trochlea must be flush with the femoral anterior cortex.

The offset guide tip is placed on the anterodistal part of the notch. The distance between the drill and guide tip never goes below 5 mm to prevent cartilage damage. Thereafter, a high-speed burr is used to remove the cancellous bone bridges between the tunnels. The guide, equipped with a cartilage palpator set at 5 mm, is used to determine the thickness of the bone resection and avoid crossing the trochlea or producing cartilage injuries inflicted by heat.

The whole trochlea is thus flexible and can be shaped without being fractured. An osteochondral cut is done following the new trochlear design. More cancellous bone could be then removed from the central metaphyseal part toward the notch, below the planned trochlear groove, to make the deepest part of the groove flush with the anterior cortex.

When trochlear deepening is considered satisfactory, a 145° Polyethylene Pusher is used to apply light pressure and mold the flap to the underlying cancellous bone bed. The lateral/medial facet external margins of the planned trochlear groove might be osteotomized to improve the amount of correction and allow greater molding. The new trochlear facets should be perfectly flush with the anterior femoral cortex proximally. The amount of deepening might be again adjusted with the motorized burr. Thin pieces of bone graft saved from the initial strip harvested with the osteotome might be placed under the lateral facet to support it in a raised position with the aim of decreasing the sulcus angle.

Once the correction obtained is adequate, the new trochlear facets are fixed with 1 absorbable anchor with 2 sutures (number 2) placed at the top of the notch. Both ends of each suture are then fixed at the proximal lateral and proximal medial (trochlear facets) bone margins of the corresponding facet with a knotless anchor. The facets are therefore compressed as the sutures are tensioned (**Fig. 5**).

Patellar tracking is then tested. The periarticular periosteum and synovial tissues are then sutured along the osteochondral margin. The associated procedures, such as

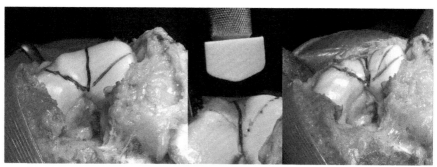

Preoperative   **Pusher 145°**   **Postoperative**

Fig. 5. From preoperative to postoperative view after deepening trochleoplasty.

tibial tuberosity medialization and/or distalization, are performed; then, the lateral retinaculum is cut or lengthened, and the last procedure done is the MPFL reconstructions.

As said, the new position of the trochlear groove is related to the preoperative TT-TG value: lateral positioning reduces the TT-TG distance by performing a proximal realignment. Therefore, in cases whereby the sulcus deepening trochleoplasty brings the TT-TG within the upper limit, the TT medialization might be not necessary. The final position of the groove is right in the middle of the femoral anatomic axis, 6° from the mechanical femoral axis.

Sulcus deepening trochleoplasty has 3 functions while treating patients with trochlear dysplasia: it modifies the trochlear shape with a central groove and oblique medial and lateral facets; it decreases the patellofemoral joint reaction force by reducing the supratrochlear prominence (spur); and it might reduce the TT-TG value.

Follow-Up and Rehabilitation

The patients are followed up radiologically and clinically. At 6 weeks postoperatively, anteroposterior, true lateral, and axial view at 30° of flexion are evaluated. At 6 months, a CT scan is obtained to evaluate the correction.

The sulcus deepening trochleoplasty procedure by itself allows full weight-bearing and no range-of-motion (ROM) limitation. Joint movement facilitates osteochondral healing and shaping the newly formed trochlea. The protocol described hereafter must be used with patients undergoing only the sulcus deepening trochleoplasty. Continuous passive motion is started the first day. If a TT osteotomy is added, full weight-bearing is allowed with an extension brace for 30 days, and ROM is limited to 100° until the 30 days as well.

During the first part of rehabilitation (first 6 weeks), full weight-bearing is allowed, without ROM limitation or a brace. Patients are therefore encouraged to perform exercise to gradually restore full ROM as tolerated, in addition to the classic protocol to reactivate and strengthen the quadriceps and hamstring muscles. Forced and painful postures should be avoided during the first phase.

After 45 days, closed-chain muscle strengthening and weight-bearing proprioception exercises are started. This includes cycling with no resistance and aquatic activities. Weight-bearing proprioception exercises are started first in bipodal and then in monopodal stance.

The third phase (3–6 months) involves a gradual return to sport: running (beginning on a straight line and then with changing directions), plyometrics, and so forth.

Sports on a recreational or competitive level might be resumed after 6 to 8 months.

Results and complications

Scientific studies related to this topic are not uniform in terms of type of trochleoplasty and associated procedures performed, inclusion criteria used, clinical outcomes measured, and the presence/absence of previous surgery. The highest clinical outcomes are demonstrated in patients with objective patellar instability, high-grade trochlear dysplasia (type B or D), and when all other anomalies that increase the risk of instability are treated simultaneously.

Generally, this procedure leads to improvements in clinical outcomes and a high rate of subjective satisfaction with a low risk of recurrence of dislocation. Among the most common complaints are a decreased postoperative ROM and pain worsening. Debated is whether this procedure has a role in patellafemoral osteoarthritis development.

Trochlear necrosis, cartilage injury, incongruence with the patella, and hypercorrection or hypocorrection are among the potential complications.

Schottle and colleagues[16] evaluated cartilage cell viability and flap healing by performing biopsies in 3 patients after trochleoplasty, outlining a low risk of cartilage damage.

Recurrence of dislocation

Instability recurrence is very rare and is more likely to be due to missed associated risk factors (patella alta, TT-TG, tilt value). The meta-analysis by Zaffagnini and colleagues[17] evaluated clinical outcomes of MPFL reconstruction with or without trochleoplasty in patients affected by trochlear dysplasia. No statistically significant differences were found in the overall redislocation rate of MPFL surgery with and without trochleoplasty.

However, they outlined that in the case of severe trochlear dysplasia (STD), the redislocation rate is lower when trochleoplasty is performed in combination with MPFL surgery.

Balcarek and colleagues[18] in their systematic review confirmed that in patients with both patellar instability and STD, trochleoplasty plus extensor mechanism balancing led to a decreased risk of subsequent postoperative redislocation/subluxation compared with simple MPFL reconstruction.

Dejour and colleagues[19] presented the outcomes of 22 patients (24 knees) with a mean follow-up of 66 months, undergoing a sulcus-deepening trochleoplasty during the period 1993 to 2006 for failure of previous patellofemoral instability surgery with persistent patellar dislocation. Among those patients, 29.1% had type B and 70.9% had type D trochlear dysplasia. After the trochleoplasty, no patient had a recurrence of dislocation up to the last follow-up. Pain decreased, and apprehension sign was negative in 72% and 75% of cases. Mean (rate) preoperative and at latest follow-up postoperative Kujala score was 44 (25–73) and 81 (53–100).

Ntagiopoulos and colleagues[12] evaluated retrospectively 27 patients (31 knees) undergoing trochleoplasty, without any previous surgery, from September 1993 to September 2006. No cases of stiffness or recurrence were observed. Apprehension signs remained positive in 19.3% of the cases, and patellar tracking was normal in all cases. The mean preoperative and postoperative International Knee Documentation Committee scores were 51 (range, 25–80) and 82 (range, 40–100) ($P<.001$), respectively, whereas the mean Kujala score improved from a preoperative 59 (range, 28–81) to 87 (range, 49–100) postoperatively ($P<.001$).

Stiffness

Postoperative stiffness is one of the main complications, sometimes requiring manipulation under anesthesia or arthroscopic arthrolysis.[10] The meta-Analysis by

Zaffagnini and colleagues[17] showed that the addition of the trochleoplasty to MPFL reconstruction for the treatment of STD might lead to a higher risk of postoperative ROM limitation compared with only MPFL reconstruction.

Blond and Haugegaard[20] followed 29 knees with trochlear dysplasia grade B or more, undergoing arthroscopic deepening trochleoplasty, for more than 12 months. No complications, redislocations, or arthrofibrosis was recorded. The median preoperative and postoperative Kujala scores (range) were 64 (12–90) and 95 (47–100), respectively. They therefore concluded that the use of arthroscopic deepening trochleoplasty is safe and reproducible.

Song and colleagues[21] evaluated patients with STD undergoing trochleoplasty or nontrochleoplasty surgical procedures. The first group showed inferior outcomes in terms of ROM.

Satisfaction

Verdonk and colleagues [22] were one of the first investigators outlining the results with sulcus deepening trochleoplasty. Although most patients scored fair and/or poor on an objective scoring system, 77% of patients achieved good to very good subjective results. Therefore, although the results were not perfect, the patients were satisfied with the procedure.

Donell and colleagues[23] reported the early results of 15 consecutive patients (17 knees) with a minimum follow-up of 1 year undergoing sulcus deepening trochleoplasty. Patellar tracking became normal in 11 knees and had a slight J-shape in 6 knees. Mild residual apprehension was present in 7 knees. Seven patients were very satisfied; 6 patients were satisfied, and 2 patients were disappointed. The mean Kujala score improved from 48 to 75. Three patients returned to full sports, and 8 patients required further operations.

Carstensen and colleagues[24] evaluated clinical outcomes of 40 patients (44 knees) with a minimum follow-up of 2 years undergoing trochleoplasty and MPFL reconstruction for STD (type B and/or D). Eight knees developed arthrofibrosis, and the overall reoperation rate was 27.3%. Patients reported a high satisfaction rate (mean 9.1 of 10). All patients returned to work, and 84.8% returned to sport. No significant radiographic patellofemoral osteoarthritis progression was outlined after surgery.

Lutz and colleagues[25] showed that despite the complexity and invasiveness, combined bony (trochlea and/or tibial tuberosity) procedures with MPFL reconstruction resulted in a low redislocation rate and improved both physical and sexual activity and quality of life compared with values reported after isolated MPFL reconstruction.

According to the systematic review by Longo and colleagues,[26] the Dejour V-shaped deepening trochleoplasty showed the highest mean Kujala postoperative score (79.3) compared with other trochleoplasty techniques.

Pain

Controversial is this procedure's efficacy in decreasing patellafemoral pain. Faruqui and colleagues[27] highlighted a higher risk of postoperative pain. All 6 of the patients undergoing the trochleoplasty were satisfied with their postoperative outcome with no recurrent instability events. However, 4 of the 6 patients reported anterior knee pain. Beaufils and colleagues[10] stated that in STD, the trochleoplasty procedure might lead to residual mild anterior knee pain. von Knoch and colleagues[28] evaluated the clinical outcomes of 38 consecutive patients (45 knees) undergoing trochleoplasty, with a mean follow-up of 8.3 years. None had recurrence of dislocation. However, patellofemoral pain, present preoperatively in only 35 knees, became worse in 15

(33.4%), remained unchanged in 4 (8.8%), and improved in 22 (49%). Four knees that had no pain preoperatively (8.8%) continued to have no pain.

Rouanet and colleagues[29] followed 34 sulcus deepening trochleoplasties for 15 years. Patients were satisfied and had occasional pain in 65% and 53% of the cases, respectively.

Osteoarthritis

Debated is the relationship between osteoarthritis, patellofemoral instability, and trochleoplasty. High-grade trochlear dysplasia leading to abnormal kinematics might increase the risk of patellofemoral osteoarthritis.[30] Whether patients with patellofemoral instability are more prone to develop osteoarthritis and whether trochleoplasty increases or protects from cartilage degeneration are not still defined clearly.[31]

Longo and colleagues[26] in their systematic review compared the 3 most popular trochleoplasty techniques (sulcus deepening trochleoplasty among them), stating that those are associated with improved stability and function and a relatively low rate of osteoarthritis and pain. von Knoch and colleagues[28] showed at mean follow-up of 8.3 years a development of patellofemoral degenerative changes in 30% of the knees treated with trochleoplasty. In Ntagiopoulos and colleagues,[12] none of the 27 patients (31 knees) had radiographic evidence of patellofemoral arthritis at the latest follow-up. Song and colleagues[21] compared the clinical outcomes between patients undergoing trochleoplasty or nontrochleoplasty procedures in treating patellar instability caused by STD (Dejour type B to D). The trochleoplasty group showed a lower rate of both redislocation and patellofemoral osteoarthritis (Iwano grade 2 or greater) progression.

Rouanet and colleagues[29] evaluated the long-term clinical outcomes and radiological rate of patellafemoral osteoarthritis in 34 sulcus-deepening trochleoplasties. No recurrent objective instability was observed. The mean Kujala and international knee society scores increased from 55 (13–75) and 127 (54–184) to 76 (51–94) and 152.4 (66–200), respectively. Functional outcomes were significantly better for sulcus deepening trochleoplasty treating dysplasia with supratrochlear spurs. Ten cases of preoperative patellofemoral osteoarthritis were identified (all cases with < Iwano 2), whereas at the final follow-up, osteoarthritis was present in 33/34 of cases, with 20 cases (65%) having more than Iwano grade 2. The investigators concluded this procedure should be limited to severe dysplasia with supratrochlear spurs and does not prevent patellofemoral osteoarthritis.

SUMMARY

Sulcus deepening trochleoplasty is a demanding procedure, having specific and selective indications: for example, patients with types B and D trochlear dysplasia, in which the prominence of the trochlea (supratrochlear spur) is important; recurrent patellar dislocation; and maltracking. It should be avoided in cases of patellofemoral osteoarthritis, open growth plates, and pain with no history of dislocations.

This procedure is highly effective in restoring patellofemoral stability and satisfying the patients. However, one must be aware of the risks of continuing residual pain and ROM limitation, and that the development of patellofemoral osteoarthritis is not predictable.

This procedure has the advantage of treating the cause at the base of instability. It modifies the trochlear shape with a central groove and oblique medial and lateral facets; it decreases the patellofemoral joint reaction force by reducing the trochlear prominence (spur) and might reduce the TT-TG value.

DISCLOSURE

E. Giovannetti de Sanctis and G. Mesnard have nothing to disclose. D.H. Dejour claims royalties from ARTHREX.

REFERENCES

1. Dejour DH. The patellofemoral joint and its historical roots: the Lyon School of Knee Surgery. Knee Surg Sports Traumatol Arthrosc 2013;21(7):1482–94.
2. Malghem J, Maldague B. Patellofemoral joint: 30 degrees axial radiograph with lateral rotation of the leg. Radiology 1989;170(2):566–7.
3. Maldague B, Malghem J. [Significance of the radiograph of the knee profile in the detection of patellar instability. Preliminary report]. Rev Chir Orthop Reparatrice Appar Mot 1985;71(Suppl 2):5–13.
4. Wiberg G. Roentgenographic and anatomic studies on the femoropatellar joint. Acta Orthop Scand 1941;12:319–410.
5. Dejour D, Saggin P. The sulcus deepening trochleoplasty-the Lyon's procedure. Int Orthop 2010;34(2):311–6.
6. Dejour D, Le Coultre B. Osteotomies in patello-femoral instabilities. Sports Med Arthrosc Rev 2007;15(1):39–46.
7. Ihara H. Double-contrast CT arthrography of the cartilage of the patellofemoral joint. Clin Orthop Relat Res 1985;198:50–5.
8. Carrillon Y, Abidi H, Dejour D, et al. Patellar instability: assessment on MR images by measuring the lateral trochlear inclination-initial experience. Radiology 2000; 216(2):582–5.
9. Staubli HU, Durrenmatt U, Porcellini B, et al. Anatomy and surface geometry of the patellofemoral joint in the axial plane. J Bone Joint Surg Br 1999;81(3):452–8.
10. Beaufils P, Thaunat M, Pujol N, et al. Trochleoplasty in major trochlear dysplasia: current concepts. Sports Med Arthrosc Rehabil Ther Technol 2012;4:7.
11. Schottle PB, Fucentese SF, Pfirrmann C, et al. Trochleaplasty for patellar instability due to trochlear dysplasia: a minimum 2-year clinical and radiological follow-up of 19 knees. Acta Orthop 2005;76(5):693–8.
12. Ntagiopoulos PG, Byn P, Dejour D. Midterm results of comprehensive surgical reconstruction including sulcus-deepening trochleoplasty in recurrent patellar dislocations with high-grade trochlear dysplasia. Am J Sports Med 2013;41(5): 998–1004.
13. Masse Y. [Trochleoplasty. Restoration of the intercondylar groove in subluxations and dislocations of the patella]. Rev Chir Orthop Reparatrice Appar Mot 1978; 64(1):3–17.
14. Dejour H, Walch G, Neyret P, et al. [Dysplasia of the femoral trochlea]. Rev Chir Orthop Reparatrice Appar Mot 1990;76(1):45–54.
15. Brittberg M, Winalski CS. Evaluation of cartilage injuries and repair. J Bone Joint Surg Am 2003;85-A(Suppl 2):58–69.
16. Schottle PB, Schell H, Duda G, et al. Cartilage viability after trochleoplasty. Knee Surg Sports Traumatol Arthrosc 2007;15(2):161–7.
17. Zaffagnini S, Previtali D, Tamborini S, et al. Recurrent patellar dislocations: trochleoplasty improves the results of medial patellofemoral ligament surgery only in severe trochlear dysplasia. Knee Surg Sports Traumatol Arthrosc 2019;27(11): 3599–613.
18. Balcarek P, Rehn S, Howells NR, et al. Results of medial patellofemoral ligament reconstruction compared with trochleoplasty plus individual extensor apparatus balancing in patellar instability caused by severe trochlear dysplasia: a

systematic review and meta-analysis. Knee Surg Sports Traumatol Arthrosc 2017; 25(12):3869–77.

19. Dejour D, Byn P, Ntagiopoulos PG. The Lyon's sulcus-deepening trochleoplasty in previous unsuccessful patellofemoral surgery. Int Orthop 2013;37(3):433–9.

20. Blond L, Haugegaard M. Combined arthroscopic deepening trochleoplasty and reconstruction of the medial patellofemoral ligament for patients with recurrent patella dislocation and trochlear dysplasia. Knee Surg Sports Traumatol Arthrosc 2014;22(10):2484–90.

21. Song GY, Hong L, Zhang H, et al. Trochleoplasty versus nontrochleoplasty procedures in treating patellar instability caused by severe trochlear dysplasia. Arthroscopy 2014;30(4):523–32.

22. Verdonk R, Jansegers E, Stuyts B. Trochleoplasty in dysplastic knee trochlea. Knee Surg Sports Traumatol Arthrosc 2005;13(7):529–33.

23. Donell ST, Joseph G, Hing CB, et al. Modified Dejour trochleoplasty for severe dysplasia: operative technique and early clinical results. Knee 2006;13(4): 266–73.

24. Carstensen SE, Feeley SM, Burrus MT, et al. Sulcus deepening trochleoplasty and medial patellofemoral ligament reconstruction for patellofemoral instability: a 2-year study. Arthroscopy 2020;36(8):2237–45.

25. Lutz PM, Winkler PW, Rupp MC, et al. Complex patellofemoral reconstruction leads to improved physical and sexual activity in female patients suffering from chronic patellofemoral instability. Knee Surg Sports Traumatol Arthrosc 2021; 29(9):3017–24.

26. Longo UG, Vincenzo C, Mannering N, et al. Trochleoplasty techniques provide good clinical results in patients with trochlear dysplasia. Knee Surg Sports Traumatol Arthrosc 2018;26(9):2640–58.

27. Faruqui S, Bollier M, Wolf B, et al. Outcomes after trochleoplasty. Iowa Orthop J 2012;32:196–206.

28. von Knoch F, Bohm T, Burgi ML, et al. Trochleaplasty for recurrent patellar dislocation in association with trochlear dysplasia. A 4- to 14-year follow-up study. J Bone Joint Surg Br 2006;88(10):1331–5.

29. Rouanet T, Gougeon F, Fayard JM, et al. Sulcus deepening trochleoplasty for patellofemoral instability: a series of 34 cases after 15 years postoperative follow-up. Orthop Traumatol Surg Res 2015;101(4):443–7.

30. Amis AA, Oguz C, Bull AM, et al. The effect of trochleoplasty on patellar stability and kinematics: a biomechanical study in vitro. J Bone Joint Surg Br 2008;90(7): 864–9.

31. Maenpaa H, Lehto MU. Patellofemoral osteoarthritis after patellar dislocation. Clin Orthop Relat Res 1997;339:156–62.

Medial Patellofemoral Ligament Reconstruction
Tips and Tricks to Get It Right

Gregory Anderson, MD[a],*, David R. Diduch, MD[b]

KEYWORDS

- Patellar instability • MPFL • Reconstruction • Technique

KEY POINTS

- Graft choice is almost never the cause of failure, with both autografts and allografts being sufficiently strong.
- The patellar attachment of the medial patellofemoral ligament is on the upper 50% of the medial patella.
- A perfect lateral radiograph intraoperatively is crucial for identifying Schottle's point, the femoral medial patellofemoral ligament attachment, and most important part of the case.
- Once Schottle's point is identified, isometry should be tested with the graft around the femoral pin.
- The phrases "high and tight" and "low and loose" can help to troubleshoot femoral graft placement intraoperatively when isometry is not present.

The medial patellofemoral ligament (MPFL) is known to be the primary soft tissue restraint against lateral translation of the patella during the first 30° of knee flexion.[1,2] After the 30° of flexion, the patella engages the trochlear groove, which provides stability throughout the remainder of the flexion arc. When the patella undergoes a lateral dislocation, the MPFL has been shown to tear at least 87% of the time, leading to the loss of this primary soft tissue stabilizer. Historically, attempts were made to repair the ruptured ligament; however, that practice has now fallen out of favor owing to inconsistency in the results and late failures.[3,4] Reconstruction of the MPFL has largely replaced repair of the ligament. This article focuses on tips and tricks to reconstruct the MPFL both in preoperative planning and intraoperative troubleshooting. An emphasis is placed on graft selection, patellar attachment, and the all-important femoral attachment.

[a] University of Virginia, 5 Trendland Cove, Sandy, UT 84092, USA; [b] Department of Orthopaedic Surgery, University of Virginia, Charlottesville, VA 22903, USA
* Corresponding author.
E-mail address: greganderson14@gmail.com

Clin Sports Med 41 (2022) 89–96
https://doi.org/10.1016/j.csm.2021.07.003
0278-5919/22/© 2021 Elsevier Inc. All rights reserved.

TECHNIQUE CONSIDERATIONS
Graft Selection

There are many options for graft choice, including a hamstring autograft or allograft, quadriceps tendon, adductor tendon, and synthetic grafts. The tensile strength required for the MPFL to fail is only about 208 N of force.[1] As such, most grafts provide a minimum of that tensile strength and are very rarely the cause of failure. Having said that, it is our preferred technique to use gracilis autograft. Its strength exceeds the native MPFL and there is no extra cost for an allograft.[5,6] Many surgeons prefer allograft semitendinosus based on even greater size and strength and to minimize incisions for autograft harvest. The extra-articular location of the MPFL is favorable for healing of an allograft.

Patellar Attachment

The MPFL attaches on the proximal one-half to two-thirds of the medial aspect of the patella and is about 17 mm wide.[7] Although this factor is important, it is not nearly as critical as the correct femoral attachment.[8–10] In general, the options include using 1 tail of the graft versus 2 tails, although 2 tails do cover more of the native patellar insertion.

There are various acceptable methods for patellar fixation including suture anchors (**Fig. 1**), interference screws, transpatellar sutures, suspensory techniques, and bone tunnels.[11–14] That being said, full-width transverse patellar drill holes do have an increased fracture risk and should be avoided. This was seen using larger diameter (4.5-mm) tunnels[15]; however, small (3.2-mm), short, oblique patellar tunnels for patellar fixation have been shown not to increase fracture risk or complications in MPFL reconstruction.[16]

Our preferred technique involves using 2 short, oblique drill holes that are 3.2 mm in diameter. The graft is looped through the patella and sterile mineral oil is used to assist with tight graft passage. This practice saves the expense of suture anchors and eliminates concern for anchor pull out. The graft is passed between the capsule and the medial retinaculum toward the femoral attachment (**Fig. 2**).

If one does consider suture anchor fixation, consideration should be given to using nonabsorbable anchors. The medially directed forces on the graft may be problematic if the graft is merely adhered to the side of the patella and the anchors eventually dissolve. Also, the surgeon should be aware that most anchors were designed for more dense bone, such as in the glenoid, and the surgeon should be sure to test the anchor's security.

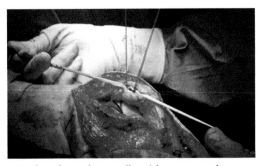

Fig. 1. Cortical fixation of graft on the patella with suture anchors.

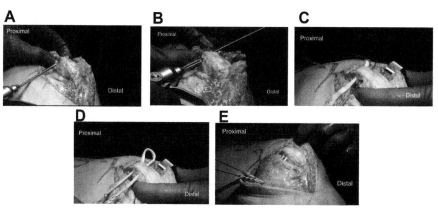

Fig. 2. Short oblique tunnel fixation. (*A*) A 3.2-mm drill bit is used to drill short oblique tunnels in the upper half of the medial patella. (*B*) A second tunnel is drilled parallel to the first with the 3.2-mm drill bit. Placing the beath pin in the first tunnel helps avoid tunnel convergence. (*C*) The beath pin is then used to pass the graft through the short, oblique patellar tunnel. (*D*) Here the graft can be seen looping through the patellar tunnels. (*E*) The graft is shown here being shuttled in between layers 2 and 3 of the medial knee toward the femoral attachment.

Femoral Attachment

The femoral attachment during an MPFL reconstruction is arguably the most important aspect of the procedure and also carries with it more controversy when compared with the patellar attachment.[4] The goal of the MPFL femoral attachment should be to restore the disrupted anatomy to minimize complications.[4,17] As such, the correct femoral graft location is key for graft isometry and incorrect position is a risk for surgical failure or chondral damage owing to increased pressure.[3,10,17,18]

The most critical tool for finding the correct femoral attachment of the graft is the use of intraoperative fluoroscopy. This step is vital to be able to localize Schottle's point.[19,20] Although this is a radiographic landmark, it is remarkably reliable for estimating the anatomic insertion of the MPFL, which can then be confirmed through cycling the knee to observe graft behavior, as described elsewhere in this article.

The femoral attachment can be located by understanding reference lines on a perfect lateral of the distal femur (**Fig. 3**).

1. A line continued distally from the posterior femoral cortex
2. Two perpendicular lines: One at the posterior aspect of Blumensaat's line, and one at the transition of the curve of the posterior femoral condyle to the posterior cortex
3. Schottle's point rests on the posterior cortical line between the perpendicular lines

This technique is a well-established and commonly used. It is very important to emphasize once again the importance of a perfect lateral radiograph of the knee for accuracy of the femoral insertion. Although this technique is our preferred technique, other methods for defining the femoral attachment exist including dividing the distal femur into percentages based off of the anterior and posterior dimension of the distal femur.[21] There are small variations in the anatomy of the distal femur that exist so intraoperative adjustments are occasionally needed and the surgeon should understand how to adapt accordingly.[21,22]

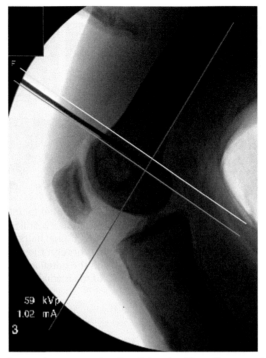

Fig. 3. Schottle's point can be seen at the tip of the pin. Three lines are drawn to help iden-tify this point. The *red line* is continued distally along the posterior cortex of the femur. The *yellow line* is drawn perpendicular to the *red line* at the transition of the curve of the pos-terior femoral condyle to the posterior cortex. Finally, the *green line* is drawn perpendicular to the *red line* at the posterior most aspect of Blumensaat's line. Schottle's point rests on the posterior cortical line between the perpendicular lines.

Once the proper attachment site is identified with fluoroscopy, the beath pin should be advanced proximally and anteriorly away from the posterior cortex. Next, the knee needs to be cycled through a full range of motion while observing the graft behavior. If the patella fixation is done first, the graft can be looped around the femoral pin at the desired attachment point. If the graft tension will be set on the patella after the femur, a suture can be used as a surrogate for the graft to observe behavior through an arc of motion. The knee is taken through a range of motion to verify that the graft remains isometric. It is important to understand normal length–tension relationships for the native MPFL to trouble shoot in the operating room. Depending on the study, the MPFL is mostly isometric from 0° to 70° or 0° to 110° of knee flexion.[21,23] Beyond this degree of flexion, the native MPFL actually becomes less taught because the pa-tella is deeply contained by the trochlea. Also, in hyperextension the MPFL becomes slightly tighter.

Unfortunately, even with restoration of the anatomic femoral insertion based off of the perfect lateral radiograph, the distal femur may have anatomic variations, which necessitate the fine-tuning of the femoral attachment. Burrus and colleagues[24] evalu-ated what intraoperative adjustments can be made if a lack of isometry is noted with the femoral attachment (**Fig. 4**).

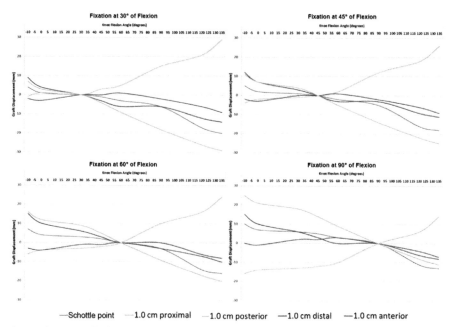

Fig. 4. These graphs from Burrus and colleagues depict different femoral attachments with the model MPFL fixed at different angles. Of note, the top left graft shows the difference of fixation with the knee at 30° of flexion. The recommended position for femoral fixation is 30° to 45° of flexion. (*From* Burrus, Werner, Conte, Diduch, Troubleshooting the Femoral Attachment During Medial Patellofemoral Ligament Reconstruction: Location, Location, Location, Orthopedic Journal of Sports Medicine (epub January, 2015, 2325967115569198. Copyright OJSM. doi:10.1177/2325967115569198). With Permission.)

1. If the graft is too tight when the knee is brought into flexion, then the femoral attachment is too proximal or high, that is, "high and tight."
2. If the graft is too loose when the knee is brought into flexion, then the femoral attachment is too distal or low, that is, "low and loose."

These simple phrases of high and tight and low and loose can aid in intraoperative adjustments to help avoid complications. If the surgeon is going to err, it should be on the side of being loose in flexion. The rationale being that in deeper flexion the trochlear groove is the primary patellar stabilizer, so a loose graft will not destabilize the patella. In contrast, a tight graft can lead to graft rupture, lack of flexion, or pressure induced chondral damage.

Knee Flexion Angle

The distal femur is not a perfect circle but is cam shaped, which suggests the importance of the correct angle for graft fixation. Multiple graft fixation angles have been described ranging from 0° to 90°.[4,9,17,18,25] Having said that, the most common degrees of flexion described are between 30 and 60°. Burrus and colleagues[24] found that fixing the graft beyond 90° of flexion magnifies incorrect femoral tunnel position and that the most isometric range of motion was noted between 0° and 70°. Fixing the graft with the knee at 0° to 30° of flexion provides the possibility of overtightening the graft because the patella does not have any bony restraints owing to a lack of trochlear engagement. Our recommended technique is to tighten the graft at between 30° and 45° of flexion. You want just enough flexion that the patella is engaged in the trochlea. This strategy will help to minimize any harmful effects of a poorly placed femoral tunnel and avoids the overtensioning that can occur when the patella is not yet engaged in the trochlea.

Care should be taken not to overtension the graft because it only needs about 2 N of force.[9,26] Overtension results in loss of flexion, medial patellar subluxation, and increased joint forces, and can lead to chondrosis.[4,9,17,18,25] When assessing the patellar translation intraoperatively, the surgeon should be able to translate the patella between 1 and 2 quadrants laterally.[27]

There are various ways of actually fixing the graft to the femur including an interference screw or a suture anchor. Our preferred technique is to create a 7-mm tunnel, pull through both graft tails, and place a 7-mm interference screw for a line to line fit.

SUMMARY

Although there are various components to an MPFL reconstruction, the femoral attachment can be the most difficult part to do correctly. Incorrect placement of the femoral attachment of the MPFL graft can lead to well-studied complications. These complications can be avoided, however, by following radiographic guidelines to find the isometric point as well as making intraoperative adjustments. The phrases of high and tight and low and loose are simple concepts that a surgeon can use to make these adjustments and avoid improper graft placement.

CLINICS CARE POINTS

- Use intra-operative fluoroscopy for femoral tunnel placement.
- The worst femoral tunnel placement is too proximal - the graft tightens with flexion and can result in loss of flexion or graft rupture.
- Fix the graft at roughly 30-45 degrees of flexion - just enough to center the patella in the trochlea.
- Don't over tighten the graft - this is the easiest mistake to make.

DISCLOSURE

G. Anderson has no relevant disclosures. D. Diduch has an institutional grant and research support from Zimmer, Aesculap, and Moximed. He is a consultant for Depuy Mitek and receives royalties from Smith and Nephew.

REFERENCES

1. Amis AA, Firer P, Mountney J, et al. Anatomy and biomechanics of the medial patellofemoral ligament. Knee 2003;10(3):215–20.
2. Bicos J, Fulkerson JP, Amis A. Current concepts review: the medial patellofemoral ligament. Am J Sports Med 2007;35(3):484–92.
3. Camp CL, Krych AJ, Dahm DL, et al. Medial patellofemoral ligament repair for recurrent patellar dislocation. Am J Sports Med 2010;38(11):2248–54.
4. Sanchis-Alfonso V. Guidelines for medial patellofemoral ligament reconstruction in chronic lateral patellar instability. J Am Acad Orthop Surg 2014;22(3):175–82.

5. Hamner DL, Brown CH, Steiner ME, et al. Hamstring tendon grafts for reconstruction of the anterior cruciate ligament: biomechanical evaluation of the use of multiple strands and tensioning techniques. J Bone Joint Surg Am 1999;81(4): 549–57.
6. Caplan N, Kader DF. Biomechanical analysis of human ligament grafts used in knee-ligament repairs and reconstructions. Class Pap Orthop 2014;145–7.
7. Barnett AJ, Howells NR, Burston BJ, et al. Radiographic landmarks for tunnel placement in reconstruction of the medial patellofemoral ligament. Knee Surg SportsTraumatol Arthrosc 2012;20(1):2380-2384.
8. Steensen RN, Dopirak RM, McDonald WG. The anatomy and isometry of the medial patellofemoral ligament: implications for reconstruction. Am J Sports Med 2004;32(6):1509–13.
9. Stephen JM, Kaider D, Lumpaopong P, et al. The effect of femoral tunnel position and graft tension on patellar contact mechanics and kinematics after medial patellofemoral ligament reconstruction. Am J Sports Med 2014;42(2):364–72.
10. Tateishi T, Tsuchiya M, Motosugi N, et al. Graft length change and radiographic assessment of femoral drill hole position for medial patellofemoral ligament reconstruction. Knee Surg Sports Traumatol Arthrosc 2011;19(3):400–7.
11. Mariani PP, Liguori L, Cerullo G, et al. Arthroscopic patellar reinsertion of the MPFL in acute patellar dislocations. Knee Surg Sports Traumatol Arthrosc 2011;19(4):628–33.
12. Schöttle PB, Hensler D, Imhoff AB. Anatomical double-bundle MPFL reconstruction with an aperture fixation. Knee Surg Sports Traumatol Arthrosc 2010;18(2): 147–51.
13. Siebold R, Chikale S, Sartory N, et al. Hamstring graft fixation in MPFL reconstruction at the patella using a transosseous suture technique. Knee Surg Sports Traumatol Arthrosc 2010;18(11):1542–4.
14. Song SY, Kim IS, Chang HG, et al. Anatomic medial patellofemoral ligament reconstruction using patellar suture anchor fixation for recurrent patellar instability. Knee Surg Sports Traumatol Arthrosc 2014;22(10):2431–7.
15. Schiphouwer L, Rood A, Tigchelaar S, et al. Complications of medial patellofemoral ligament reconstruction using two transverse patellar tunnels. Knee Surg Sports Traumatol Arthrosc 2017;25(1):245–50.
16. Deasey MJ, Moran TE, Lesevic M, et al. Small, short, oblique patellar tunnels for patellar fixation do not increase fracture risk or complications in MPFL reconstruction: a retrospective cohort study. Orthop J Sport Med 2020;8(10):1–7.
17. Elias JJ, Cosgarea AJ. Technical errors during medial patellofemoral ligament reconstruction could overload medial patellofemoral cartilage: a computational analysis. Am J Sports Med 2006;34(9):1478–85.
18. Bollier M, Fulkerson J, Cosgarea A, et al. Technical failure of medial patellofemoral ligament reconstruction. Arthroscopy 2011;27(8):1153–9.
19. Redfern J, Kamath G, Burks R. Anatomical confirmation of the use of radiographic landmarks in medial patellofemoral ligament reconstruction. Am J Sports Med 2010;38(2):293–7.
20. Schöttle PB, Schmeling A, Rosenstiel N, et al. Radiographic landmarks for femoral tunnel placement in medial patellofemoral ligament reconstruction. Am J Sports Med 2007;35(5):801–4.
21. Stephen JM, Lumpaopong P, Deehan DJ, et al. The medial patellofemoral ligament: Location of femoral attachment and length change patterns resulting from anatomic and nonanatomic attachments. Am J Sports Med 2012;40(8): 1871–9.

22. Siebold R, Borbon CAV. Arthroscopic extraarticular reconstruction of the medial patellofemoral ligament with gracilis tendon autograft - surgical technique. Knee Surg Sports Traumatol Arthrosc 2012;20(7):1245–51.
23. Smirk C, Morris H. The anatomy and reconstruction of the medial patellofemoral ligament. Knee 2003;10(3):221–7.
24. Tyrrell Burrus M, Werner BC, Conte EJ, et al. Troubleshooting the femoral attachment during medial patellofemoral ligament reconstruction: location, location, location. Orthop J Sport Med 2015;3(1):1–8.
25. Thaunat M, Erasmus PJ. Management of overtight medial patellofemoral ligament reconstruction. Knee Surg Sports Traumatol Arthrosc 2009;17(5):480–3.
26. Beck P, Brown NAT, Greis PE, et al. Patellofemoral contact pressures and lateral patellar translation after medial patellofemoral ligament reconstruction. Am J Sports Med 2007;35(9):1557–63.
27. Arendt EA. Medial side patellofemoral anatomy: surgical implications in patellofemoral instability. In: Patellofemoral pain, instability, and arthritis: clinical presentation, imaging, and treatment. Springer Berlin Heidelberg; 2010. p. 149–52.

Medial Patellofemoral Ligament Reconstruction with Open Physes

Sofia Hidalgo Perea, BS[a], Sara R. Shannon[b],
Daniel W. Green, MD, MS[a],*

KEYWORDS

- Patellofemoral instability • Knee • Pediatric • MPFL • Surgical treatment
- Open physes

KEY POINTS

- Management and treatment of pediatric and adolescent patellofemoral instability (PFI) continue to evolve, and there is large variability in the surgical techniques to reconstruct the medial patellofemoral ligament (MPFL) in an immature patient.
- A variety of different physeal-sparing techniques that address the common medial soft tissue instability have been shown to be safe and effective.
- The authors' preferred techniques consist of using a double 2-limbed free hamstring autograft or allograft to reconstruct the MPFL using a femoral anchor in the epiphysis below the growth plate.

INTRODUCTION

A recent study highlighted an increase in the incidence of lateral patellar dislocations with about 23.2 per 100,000 people per year.[1] The highest incidence of the orthopedic injury was found in adolescents aged between 14 and 18 years old. At 147.4 per 100,000 people per year for that age group and no difference between sexes, it is evident that they are a high-risk group.

With such a high recurrence rate, many studies have monitored patients over the 10 years since their first-time lateral patellar dislocation. A 2017 population-based study conducted by Christensen and colleagues[2] included a mean follow-up of 12.4 years for 584 patients with a first-time lateral patellar dislocation occurring between 1990 and 2010. Of these patients, 173 patients had had ipsilateral recurrence, and 25 patients had a subsequent contralateral dislocation. At 20 years, the cumulative incidence of ipsilateral recurrence was 36.0%, whereas the cumulative incidence

[a] Department of Pediatric Orthopedics, Hospital for Special Surgery, 535 East 70th Street, New York, NY 10021, USA; [b] Department of Neuroscience, Duke University, Durham, NC, USA
* Corresponding author.
E-mail address: greendw@hss.edu

Clin Sports Med 41 (2022) 97–108
https://doi.org/10.1016/j.csm.2021.07.004
0278-5919/22/© 2021 Elsevier Inc. All rights reserved.

of contralateral dislocations was 5.4%. Their findings also commented on the prevalence of trochlear dysplasia, which describes the orthopedic condition whereby the trochlea is displastic, usually flattened, and therefore cannot properly fit the patella that would regularly rest in its groove. Trochlear dysplasia (odds ratio [OR], 18.1), patella alta (OR, 10.4), and age less than 18 years at the time of the first dislocation (OR, 2.4) were associated with recurrent ipsilateral dislocations.

Patellar instability surgical treatment has classically been indicated after a patient has suffered a second dislocation, but in individuals with numerous risk factors, surgical stabilization options may also be considered. This article reviews medial patellofemoral ligament (MPFL) reconstruction techniques that exist for skeletally immature patients.

SURGICAL INDICATIONS

Management and treatment of pediatric and adolescent PFI continue to change in the orthopedic field, and variability in surgical techniques continues to exist.

Generally, first-time dislocators who present with no risk factors for PFI are treated nonoperatively with activity modification and formal course of physical therapy, as studies have shown that acute first-time dislocations do not necessarily benefit from surgery, and those who have compared nonoperative versus operative treatment have demonstrated that functional outcomes remain equal between the 2 treatment options.[3–6] However, in a randomized trial, Bitar and colleagues[7] showed that MPFL reconstruction performed in first-time dislocators resulted in improved clinical and patient-reported outcomes when compared with patients treated nonoperatively. The operative group had no recurrent instability episodes, whereas the nonoperative group had a 35% recurrence rate and the mean Kujala score was 88.9 in comparison to 70.8 at 2-year follow-up, highlighting that more research needs to be conducted to elucidate the best treatment algorithm.

Patients who present with recurrent PFI are indicated for surgical treatment to prevent experiencing multiple events of patellofemoral instability and to prevent articular damage. The authors' preferred algorithm for PFI treatment takes into account the presence of osteochondral lesions, number of events, anatomic risk factors, and skeletal maturity (**Table 1**).[8]

MEDIAL PATELLOFEMORAL LIGAMENT RECONSTRUCTION IN SKELETALLY IMMATURE PATIENTS: PROCEDURES AND TECHNIQUES

MPFL reconstruction has become the standard of care for patients presenting with recurrent PFI. A variety of different physeal-sparing techniques that address the

---

Table 1
Indications for medial patellofemoral ligament reconstruction in the skeletally immature patient

First-time patellar dislocation if:	Recurrent patellofemoral instability:
• Osteochondral defect or loose body	• Recurrent lateral patellar dislocations
• Persistent symptoms of instability despite adequate nonoperative management	• Symptomatic obligatory dislocation in extension
• Multiple risk factors, including history of contralateral patellar dislocation/stabilization	• Fixed dislocation or obligatory dislocation in flexion (MPFL reconstruction performed in conjunction with quadricepsplasty)

medial soft tissue instability that is commonplace in these patients have been shown to be safe and effective.[9,10]

Double Bundle Hamstring Graft Using Patellar and Femoral Anchors

The authors' preferred technique consists of using a double two-limbed free hamstring autograft or allograft to reconstruct the MPFL, as previously described by Farr and Schepsis.[11] The gracilis or semitendinosis is harvested and prepared followed by the reaming of 2 short and small-diameter sockets in the superior half of the patella. The location of the epiphyseal femoral socket is confirmed on intraoperative fluoroscopy by placing a guidewire just below the distal femoral growth plate (DFGP) on the anteroposterior (AP) image and in line with the posterior femoral cortex on the lateral view similar to the radiographic landmarks described by Schöttle and colleagues[12] (**Fig. 1**). Because of the fact that the DFGP is not linear, the aperture of the DFGP socket may appear to be at or above the level of the growth plate on the lateral knee view, while clearly being below and away from the growth plate on the AP view.[13]

The use of fluoroscopic guidance when reaming the femoral socket is also encouraged, as a previous study conducted by Uppstrom and colleagues[14] demonstrated that it was an effective method to avoid physeal injury and subsequent growth disturbance. The study, which included 54 skeletally immature knees aged 13.3 ± 1.6 years, reported no statistically significant difference in leg length between operated and non-operated extremities and no evidence of physeal arrest on MRI. Moreover, the drill should be angled distally and anteriorly as previously described by Bishop and colleagues[15] to avoid physeal injury. The authors check isometrics before drilling of the socket, by placing the graft or a suture around the guidewire and to the medial edge of the patella. The doubled-over portion of the of the graft is then secured into a single femoral socket using a tenodesis screw, and the free ends of the double-ended limb of the graft are secured into 2 short patella sockets using tenodesis screws or swivel locks (**Fig. 2**).

In a study that included 23 skeletally immature patients who underwent MPFL reconstruction with a double bundle hamstring autograft, Ladenhauf and colleagues[13] demonstrated excellent clinical outcomes at mean follow-up of 16 months. Moreover, Nelitz and colleagues[16] demonstrated similar outcomes in a group of 21 skeletally

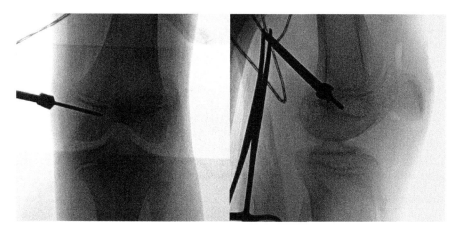

Fig. 1. The use of fluoroscopic guidance when reaming the femoral socket.

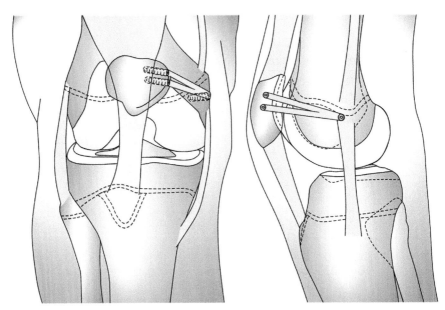

Fig. 2. Double bundle hamstring graft using patellar and femoral sockets.

immature patients; at mean follow-up of 2.8 years, the mean Kujala score was significantly higher than preoperatively (72.9 vs 92.8; $P<.1$).

A potential serious postoperative complication surgeons must watch out for when performing this technique is that of associated of iatrogenic patella fracture.[17,18] In a case report that included 5 patella fractures, Parikh and Wall[17] reported that most complications were secondary to technical factors that occurred during the index procedure. Similarly, Tanaka and colleagues[18] concluded that surgeons can avoid this error by studying the complications associated with the procedure.

Hamstring Graft with Attachment to Medial Quadriceps Tendon

Another technique that has gained popularity in the last decade involved the medial quadriceps tendon femoral ligament (MQTFL). Because of its pure soft tissue attachment into the extensor mechanism, reconstruction techniques avoid the use of drilling tunnels, which is advantageous when performing surgery on skeletally immature patients.[19] Fulkerson and Edgar[20] described this technique in 2013 and reported results similar to those of MPFL reconstruction in patients with 3-year follow-up. In this technique, the graft is secured to the adductor tubercule to reconstruct the MQTFL and obtain stabilization of the patellofemoral joint without the risk of patella fracture that MPFL reconstructions have (**Fig. 3**).[21]

Combined MPFL and MQTFL reconstruction has been shown to have favorable short-term results.[22] In a recent study, Spang and colleagues[23] reported that both MPFL and MQTFL reconstructions provided stability throughout the joint. Although MQTFL re-created native stability in a cadaver model, MPFL reconstruction was associated with increased resistance to lateral translation.

Hamstring Graft Using the Adductor Tendon as a Pulley

Another technique uses a hamstring autograft or allograft (either gracilis or semitendinosis), which is then looped around the adductor magnus tendon, which acts

Quadriceps   Vastus Medialis Obliquus
Tendon   Muscle

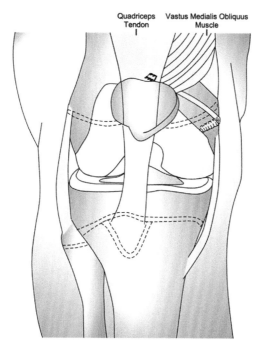

Fig. 3. Hamstring graft with attachment to medial quadriceps tendon.

as a pulley before being docked to the medial aspect of the patella (**Fig. 4**).[24] Kiran and colleagues[25] have also performed a similar but less commonly used technique using the medial collateral ligament as a pulley. They reported no recurrent episodes of dislocation or subluxation at 24 months of follow-up.

The authors utilize this technique in very young pediatric patients, especially those with a syndromic association that have weak or very small epiphyseal bone.

Pedicle Adductor Magnus Tendon: Adductor Magnus Tenodesis

Another technique for pediatric MPFL reconstruction uses a pedicled adductor magnus tendon, pedicled quadriceps tendon, or pedicled patellar tendon (**Fig. 5**). Referred to as an adductor magnus tenodesis, this technique consists of performing a tenodesis of the distal adductor magnus tendon to the medial border of the patella.[26] Malecki and colleagues[27] reported results of this technique in a cohort of children and adolescents. Although 4 patients experienced subsequent dislocations, Lysholm and Kujala scores significantly improved postoperatively ($P<.001$).

Moreover, although less often used, the pedicled quadriceps tendon or pedicled patellar tendon is also used, as they do not involve any bony procedure, avoiding physeal disturbance or patella fractures. First described by Steensen and colleagues and later refined by Goyal,[28–30] the pedicled quadriceps technique involves a partial-thickness graft from the central one-third of the patella that is docked at the medial epicondyle. Similarly, the pedicled patellar tendon technique involves the harvesting of the medial aspect of the patellar tendon. Both techniques showed better clinical outcomes and improved patient-reported outcomes when compared with nonoperative treatment.[7,16]

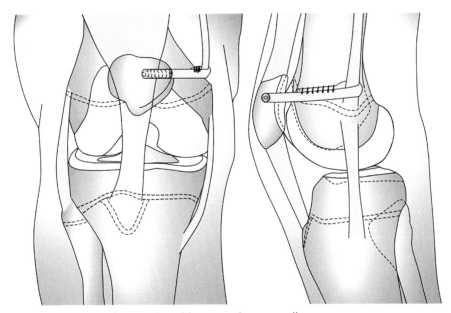

Fig. 4. Hamstring graft using the adductor tendon as a pulley.

NEED TO DO MORE? ADDITIONAL CONSIDERATIONS AND PROCEDURES
Distal Realignment

Distal realignment procedures are commonly performed on patients with a large tibial tubercle-trochlear groove (TT-TG) distance or pathologic patella alta. TT-TG measurements on axial imaging that are greater than 20 mm and a "Q angle" greater than 23° have been known to warrant correction.[31]

Tibial tubercle transfers are one of the most common forms of distal realignment in skeletally mature patients. The Fulkerson osteotomy is a type of tibial tubercle transfer involving an anterior and medial transfer of the tubercle.[32] Anteromedialization of the tibial tubercle, achieved by the Fulkerson osteotomy, helps by ensuring earlier contact between the patella and trochlea in flexion as a result of improved patella tracking.[32]

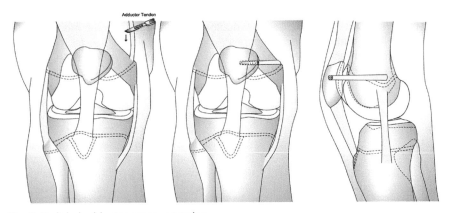

Fig. 5. Pedicled adductor magnus tendon.

Because of the risk of physeal arrest and subsequent growth disturbances, this procedure is only performed on skeletally mature patients.

In contrast, the Roux-Goldthwait procedure, an additional type of tibial tubercle transfer, is often done on skeletally immature patients, as it is considered a soft tissue procedure and decreases a large "Q angle" without threatening the physis.[33] In this realignment, the patellar tendon is vertically split, resulting in the lateral half of the tendon detaching from the tibial tuberosity. The tendon is translated and positioned medially and attached to the tibia. Trivellas and colleagues[33] recently chose a combination of a Roux-Goldthwait procedure and an allograft MPFL reconstruction to improve many of their patients' instability. These surgeries have successfully restored patella tracking and proper knee balance. Another popular realignment procedure is the Grammont procedure. It consists of a medialization of the patellar tendon and periosteum without compromising the growth plates.[34]

Distal realignments combined with MPFL reconstruction allow for increased improvement in alignment parameters, in particular, the patellar tilt and congruence angles.[35] This recent combination of techniques has allowed for highly successful outcomes in many patients, especially patients who are skeletally immature. Although MPFL reconstruction has proved to be a leading procedure for patellar instability, with the help of other procedures (**Fig. 6**), such as the Roux-Goldthwait or Grammont distal realignment and lateral retinacular release, surgeries can be even more successful for targeted patients (**Box 1**).

Patellofemoral Instability Associated with Genu Valgum

Genu valgum is a prevalent orthopedic deformity in the coronal plane of the lower extremity. This condition alters the forces on the lateral aspect of the patellofemoral joint, and if left uncorrected when performing an MPFL reconstruction, can lead to graft failure and poor clinical outcomes.[36,37]

Correction in skeletally immature patients can be achieved by growth modulation, such as implant-mediated guided growth (IMMG).[38–42] In a recent study, preliminary results of Parikh and colleagues[43] demonstrated that performing an MPFL and IMMG simultaneously could correct the angular deformity without interfering with the graft placement. Moreover, Ceroni and colleagues[44] reported that for every 1° of angular correction during distal femoral hemi-epiphysiodesis, there is a simultaneous 1-mm correction of TT-TG.

Lateral Retinacular Release or Lengthening

Lateral retinacular release and lengthening is another surgical resource used for patellofemoral instability (**Fig. 7**). Like the Roux-Goldthwait procedure, it is routinely used in conjunction with other procedures, such as MPFL reconstruction.[45] The lateral retinaculum is responsible for approximately 10% of the lateral stability of the patella.

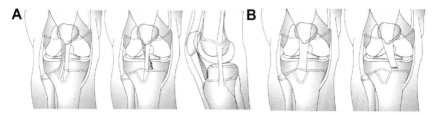

Fig. 6. Various techniques for pediatric distal realignment. (*A*) Roux-Goldthwait procedure. (*B*) Patellar tendon transfer, also referred to as the Grammont procedure.

Box 1	
Common pediatric distal realignment procedures	
Name	**Description**
Roux-Goldthwait procedure	Translation of the lateral half of the patellar tendon resulting in medial positioning attached to the tibia, providing a decreased "Q angle"
Grammont procedure	Transformation of the patellar tendon medially to the distal half of the tibia, permitting extension along the edge of the tendon

However, under immense stress, its instability can create many problems with patellar tracking and tilt.[46] The lateral retinacular release releases the lateral patellofemoral ligament and the lateral patellotibial ligament, allowing the kneecap to properly fit in the trochlear groove. Lateral lengthening as opposed to release provides further stability postoperatively; however, it is not always possible to repair the lateral retinaculum in knees with severe contracture of the lateral tissues. Finally, patellar tendon transfers are also used to correct the challenges with patellar instability discussed above. Recently, patellar tendon transfers have been performed medially to the distal half of the patella, extending along the edge of the tendon. Marteau and colleagues[47] proposed a type of patellar tendon transfer referred to as the Gracilis tendon transfer in which a gracilis muscle is transferred to the medial edge of the patella. This technique allows for proper tracking and reduces future dislocations.

Fixed or Obligatory Dislocators

Fixed dislocation refers to an irreducible lateral dislocation throughout knee range of motion. Obligatory dislocation in flexion refers to patients whose patella dislocates laterally every time their knee flexes. Fixed and obligatory dislocators present with pathologic morphologic anatomic risk factors, tight lateral structures, and often a shortened extensor mechanism that contributes to patellar instability.[48]

Different techniques have been published to guide treatment. However, because of the uncommon nature of both, there is no standard treatment algorithm in the literature. The authors' preferred technique is the stepwise lengthening of the extensor mechanism previously described by Ellsworth and colleagues[49] characterized by an extensive lateral release or lengthening, vastus lateralis lengthening, and a separate

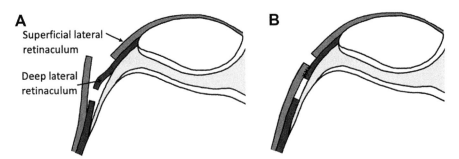

Fig. 7. Lateral retinacular lengthening. First performed by making an incision adjacent to the lateral aspect of the patella, creating an interval between the superficial oblique and deep transverse retinaculum, and transecting the deep transverse at the level of the iliotibial band (*A*). The lateral capsule is then released, and the lateral retinaculum is repaired in a lengthened position at the end of the case (*B*).

Z-lengthening of the rectus and intermedius tendon (if needed), as it permits the surgeon to preferentially lengthen the lateral aspect of the quadriceps tendon more than the medial aspect.

CLINICS CARE POINTS

Pearls	Pitfalls
• Medial patellofemoral ligament femoral insertion should be DISTAL to the growth plate	• Requires intraoperative fluoroscopy
• Consider standing alignment radiographs and treat genu valgum	• Patients with open growth plates may require additional operative time and alteration of the technique and sequence of graft placement
• Be prepared to perform an extensive lateral release and quadriceps tendon lengthening in cases of obligatory dislocation in flexion and fixed patella dislocation	
• In extremely young patients with weak epiphyseal bone, the femoral attachment of the medial patellofemoral ligament reconstruction can be moved to the distal adductor tendon	

ACKNOWLEDGMENTS

The authors would like to thank Craig Klinger for his artistic contributions.

DISCLOSURE

S.H. Perea, S.R. Shannon have nothing to disclose. Dr D.W. Green owns royalties from Pega Medical and Arthrex Inc not related to implants discussed in this review and is a paid consultant for Arthrex Inc.

REFERENCES

1. Sanders TL, Pareek A, Johnson NR, et al. Patellofemoral arthritis after lateral patellar dislocation: a matched population-based analysis. Am J Sports Med 2017;45(5):1012–7.
2. Christensen TC, Sanders TL, Pareek A, et al. Risk factors and time to recurrent ipsilateral and contralateral patellar dislocations. Am J Sports Med 2017;45(9): 2105–10.
3. Palmu S, Kallio PE, Donell ST, et al. Acute patellar dislocation in children and adolescents: a randomized clinical trial. J Bone Jonit Surg Am 2008;90(3): 463–70.
4. Apostolovic M, Vukomanovic B, Slavkovic N, et al. Acute patellar dislocation in adolescents: operative versus nonoperative treatment. Int Orthop 2011;35(10): 1483–7.
5. Erickson BJ, Mascarenhas R, Sayegh ET, et al. Does operative treatment of first-time patellar dislocations lead to increased patellofemoral stability? A systematic review of overlapping meta-analyses. Arthroscopy 2015;31(6):1207–15.
6. Sillanpää PJ, mattila V M, Mäenpää H, et al. Treatment with and without initial stabilizing surgery for primary traumatic patellar dislocation: a prospective randomized study. J Bone Joint Surg Am 2009;91(2):263–73.

7. Bitar AC, Demange MK, D'Elia CO, et al. Traumatic patellar dislocation: nonoperative treatment compared with MPFL reconstruction using patellar tendon. Am J Sports Med 2012;40(1):114–22.

8. Gausden EB, Fabricant PD, Taylor SA, et al. Medial patellofemoral reconstruction in children and adolescents. JBJS Rev 2015;3(10):1–11.

9. Haskel JD, Uppstrom TJ, Gausden EB, et al. Low risk of physeal damage from a medial patellofemoral ligament (MPFL) reconstruction technique that uses an epiphyseal socket in children. Orthop J Sport Med 2015;3(7):1.

10. Conlan T, Garth WP, Lemons JE. Evaluation of the medial soft-tissue restraints of the extensor mechanism of the knee. J Bone Joint Surg Am 1993;75(5):682–93.

11. Farr J, Schepsis AA. Reconstruction of the medial patellofemoral ligament for recurrent patellar instability. J Knee Surg 2006;19(4):307–16.

12. Schöttle P, Schmeling A, Romero J, et al. Anatomical reconstruction of the medial patellofemoral ligament using a free gracilis autograft. Arch Orthop Trauma Surg 2009;129(3):305–9.

13. Ladenhauf HN, Jones KJ, Potter HG, et al. Understanding the undulating pattern of the distal femoral growth plate: implications for surgical procedures involving the pediatric knee: a descriptive MRI study. Knee 2020;27(2):315–23.

14. Uppstrom TJ, Price M, Black S, et al. Medial patellofemoral ligament (MPFL) reconstruction technique using an epiphyseal femoral socket with fluoroscopic guidance helps avoid physeal injury in skeletally immature patients. Knee Surg Sport Traumatol Arthrosc 2019;27(11):3536–42.

15. Bishop ME, Black SR, Nguyen J, et al. A simple method of measuring the distance from the Schöttle point to the medial distal femoral physis with MRI. Orthop J Sport Med 2019;7(4). 2325967119840713.

16. Nelitz M, Dreyhaupt J, Williams SRM. Anatomic reconstruction of the medial patellofemoral ligament in children and adolescents using a pedicled quadriceps tendon graft shows favourable results at a minimum of 2-year follow-up. Knee Surg Sport Traumatol Arthrosc 2018;26(4):1210–5.

17. Parikh SN, Wall EJ. Patellar fracture after medial patellofemoral ligament surgery: a report of five cases. J Bone Joint Surg Am 2011;93(17):e97.

18. Tanaka MJ, Bollier MJ, Andrish JT, et al. Complications of medial patellofemoral ligament reconstruction: common technical errors and factors for success AAOS exhibit selection. J Bone Joint Surg Am 2012;94(12):e87.

19. Chahla J, Smigielski R, Laprade RF, et al. An updated overview of the anatomy and function of the proximal medial patellar restraints (medial patellofemoral ligament and the medial quadriceps tendon femoral ligament). Sports Med Arthrosc 2019;27(4):136–42.

20. Fulkerson JP, Edgar C. Medial quadriceps tendon-femoral ligament: surgical anatomy and reconstruction technique to prevent patella instability. Arthrosc Tech 2013;2(2):e125.

21. Joseph SM, Fulkerson JP. Medial quadriceps tendon femoral ligament reconstruction technique and surgical anatomy. Arthrosc Tech 2019;8(1):e57–64.

22. Spang RC, Tepolt FA, Paschos NK, et al. Combined reconstruction of the medial patellofemoral ligament (MPFL) and medial quadriceps tendon-femoral ligament (MQTFL) for patellar instability in children and adolescents: surgical technique and outcomes. J Pediatr Orthop 2019;39(1):e54–61.

23. Spang R, Egan J, Hanna P, et al. Comparison of patellofemoral kinematics and stability after medial patellofemoral ligament and medial quadriceps tendon–femoral ligament reconstruction. Am J Sports Med 2020;48(9):2252–9.

24. Gomes JE. Comparison between a static and a dynamic technique for medial patellofemoral ligament reconstruction. Arthroscopy 2008;24(4):430–5.
25. Kiran KR, Srikanth I, Chinnusamy L, et al. Dynamic medial patellofemoral ligament reconstruction in recurrent patellar instability: a surgical technique. Indian J Orthop 2015;49(6):630–6.
26. Avikainen V, Nikku R, Seppanen-Lehmonen T. Adductor magnus tenodesis for patellar dislocation. Technique and preliminary results. Clin Orthop Relat Res 1993;297(12):12–6.
27. Malecki K, Fabis J, Flont P, et al. The results of adductor magnus tenodesis in adolescents with recurrent patellar dislocation. Biomed Res Int 2015;2015:456858.
28. Steensen RN, Dopirak RM, Maurus PB. A simple technique for reconstruction of the medial patellofemoral ligament using a quadriceps tendon graft. Arthroscopy 2005;21(3):365–70.
29. Goyal D. Medial patellofemoral ligament reconstruction: the superficial quad technique. Am J Sports Med 2013;41(5):1022–9.
30. Nelitz M, Williams SRM. Anatomic reconstruction of the medial patellofemoral ligament in children and adolescents using a pedicled quadriceps tendon graft. Arthrosc Tech 2014;3(2):e303–8.
31. Berruto M, Ferrua P, Carimati G, et al. Patellofemoral instability: classification and imaging. Joints 2013;1(2):7–13.
32. Grimm NL, Lazarides AL, Amendola A. Tibial tubercle osteotomies: a review of a treatment for recurrent patellar instability. Curr Rev Musculoskelet Med 2018; 11(2):266–71.
33. Trivellas M, Arshi A, Beck JJ. Roux-Goldthwait and medial patellofemoral ligament reconstruction for patella realignment in the skeletally immature patient. Arthrosc Tech 2019;8(12):e1479–83.
34. Grammont PM, Latune D, Lammaire IP. Die behandlung der subluxation und luxation der kniescheibe beim kind. Technik von elmslie mit beweglichem weichteilsteil (8-jahres-ubersicht). Orthopade 1985;14(4):229–38.
35. Damasena I, Blythe M, Wysocki D, et al. Medial patellofemoral ligament reconstruction combined with distal realignment for recurrent dislocations of the patella. Am J Sports Med 2017;45(2):369–76.
36. Maquet P. Biomechanics of the knee: with application to the pathogenesis and the srugical treatment of osteoarthritis. 2nd edition. New York: Springer-Verlag; 1984.
37. Paley D. Principles of deformity correction. 1st edition. New York: Springer; 2002.
38. Brauwer V De, Moens P. Temporary hemiepiphysiodesis for idiopathic genua valga in adolescents: percutaneous transphyseal screws (PETS) versus stapling. J Pediatr Orthop 2008;28(5):549–54.
39. Castañeda P, Urquhart B, Sullivan E, et al. Hemiepiphysiodesis for the correction of angular deformity about the knee. J Pediatr Orthop 2008;28(2):188–91.
40. Redler LH, Wright ML. Surgical management of patellofemoral instability in the skeletally immature patient. J Am Acad Orthop Surg 2018;26(19):e405–15.
41. Lin KM, Thacher RR, Apostolakos JM, et al. Implant-mediated guided growth for coronal plane angular deformity in the pediatric patient with patellofemoral instability. Arthrosc Tech 2021;10(3):e913–24.
42. Saran N, Rathjen KE. Guided growth for the correction of pediatric lower limb angular deformity. J Am Acad Orthop Surg 2010;18(9):528–36.
43. Parikh SN, Redman C, Gopinathan NR. Simultaneous treatment for patellar instability and genu valgum in skeletally immature patients: a preliminary study. J Pediatr Orthop B 2019;28(2):132–8.

44. Ceroni D, Dhouib A, Merlini L, et al. Modification of the alignment between the tibial tubercle and the trochlear groove induced by temporary hemiepiphysiodesis for lower extremity angular deformities: a trigonometric analysis. J Pediatr Orthop Part B 2017;26(3):204–10.
45. Fonseca LPRM, Kawatake EH, Pochini A de C. Lateral patellar retinacular release: changes over the last ten years. Rev Bras Ortop (English Ed) 2017; 52(4):442–9.
46. Christoforakis J, Bull AMJ, Strachan RK, et al. Effects of lateral retinacular release on the lateral stability of the patella. Knee Surg Sport Traumatol Arthrosc 2006; 14(3):273–7.
47. Marteau E, Burdin P, Brilhault JM. Gracilis tendon transfer associated with distal alignment for patella alta with recurrent dislocations: an original surgical technique. Orthop Traumatol Surg Res 2011;97(4):S5.
48. Danino B, Deliberato D, Abousamra O, et al. Four-in-one extensor realignment for the treatment of obligatory or fixed, lateral patellar instability in skeletally immature knee. J Pediatr Orthop 2020;40(9):503–8.
49. Ellsworth B, Hidalgo Perea S, Green DW. Stepwise lengthening of the quadriceps extensor mechanism for severe obligatory and fixed patella dislocators. Arthrosc Tech 2021;10(5):e1327–31.

Putting it all Together
Evaluating Patellar Instability Risk Factors and Revisiting the "Menu"

Michaela I. McCarthy, MD[a], Betina B. Hinckel, MD, PhD[b,c],
Elizabeth A. Arendt, MD[a,*], Caitlin C. Chambers, MD[a,d]

KEYWORDS

- Recurrent lateral patellar dislocation • Anatomic patellar instability risk factors
- Surgical "menu" options

KEY POINTS

- The cornerstone of patient evaluation continues to be detailing all risk factors contributing to recurrent lateral patellar dislocation (LPD). However, it is not known *when* these factors must be surgically corrected and *at what numerical threshold* for best outcomes.
- Current literature supports that additive risk factors result in additive risk for recurrent LPD.
- Clinical decision making should be individualized to each patient scenario.

INTRODUCTION

The reported rate of recurrent lateral patellar dislocation (LPD) varies among studies; in a recent meta-analysis, the overall rate of recurrent LPD following first-time injury was 33.6%.[1] Recurrent LPD are associated with joint damage and loss of quality of life. Understanding the interplay of multiple risk factors for recurrent LPD is paramount in developing an appropriate treatment algorithm.[2,3] Before the advent of medial patellofemoral ligament (MPFL) reconstruction, the surgical procedures used to stabilize individual patellar instability advocated correcting each known risk factor, discussed as menu options to be chosen à la carte.[4] This is an appropriate approach to relatively simple cases of patellar instability, but the interplay of multiple recurrence risk factors makes choosing the appropriate options increasingly difficult in more complex cases. In this section, the authors discuss the risk factors that play a role in

[a] Department of Orthopedic Surgery, University of Minnesota, 2450 Riverside Ave South, Suite R200 Minneapolis, MN 55454, USA; [b] Department of Orthopaedic Surgery, William Beaumont Hospital, 10000 Telegraph Road, Suite 100, Taylor, MI 48180, USA; [c] Oakland University, Rochester, Michigan, USA; [d] TRIA Orthopedic Center, 155 Radio Drive, Woodbury, MN 55125, USA
* Corresponding author.
E-mail address: arend001@umn.edu

Clin Sports Med 41 (2022) 109–121
https://doi.org/10.1016/j.csm.2021.07.009
0278-5919/22/© 2021 Elsevier Inc. All rights reserved.

determining appropriate treatment of patients with recurrent LPD and outline their approach to the menu options for both simple and complex scenarios.

Anatomic Patellar Instability Risk Factors

The stability of the patellofemoral (PF) joint involves an intricate relationship between muscular forces, soft tissues, trochlear and patellar geometry, and limb alignment.[5] Several anatomic factors have been identified as risk factors for LPD; patella alta, trochlear dysplasia, and increased lateral quadriceps vector are the most commonly cited. However, rotational malalignment and genu valgum also play an important role.[5-7] As independent anatomic factors, trochlear dysplasia and patella alta are the most commonly encountered, with a study of primary patellar dislocations identifying these risk factors in 61% and 54% of cases, respectively.[6,8] These anatomic patellar instability (API) risk factors have been discussed at length within their individual sections of this issue and will thus be reviewed only briefly within this article. Additional risk factors not discussed elsewhere in this issue, but worthy of consideration, include skeletal immaturity, contralateral patellar dislocation, and generalized hypermobility.

The importance of these API risk factors is highlighted by their overwhelming association with patellar instability. Steensen and colleagues[6] found that 70% of individuals without a history of LPD had no API risk factors, whereas 92% of those with recurrent LPD had one or more risk factors. In addition, an increased risk of recurrence is reported in patients with younger age and open physes.[1] Patients ≤16 years old have an odds ratio (OR) for re-dislocation of 11.2 compared with individuals older than 16 years old.[9] Skeletally immature knees have a 43.3% recurrence rate compared with a 21.6% recurrence rate in skeletally mature knees ($P = .0009$).[10] Skeletal immaturity combined with trochlear dysplasia confers a 56% to 69% risk of recurrent LPD within 5 years.[10,11]

Studies have not consistently demonstrated any association between sex and recurrent LPD rates.[1,5,12] In addition, current literature does not support a significant association between sex and API risk factors, such as trochlear dysplasia, tibial torsion, tibial tubercle-trochlear groove (TT-TG) distance, and frontal mechanical axis.[5]

History of contralateral LPD increases the risk for bilateral instability (OR, 3.05–3.167), with a 62.5% recurrence rate.[9,10]

The role of generalized hypermobility in LPD is controversial. Some studies have demonstrated that hypermobility (Beighton score >6) is associated with increased rates of residual and recurrent symptoms, and lower rate of return to prior sport activity after MPFL reconstruction.[13] Conversely, another study demonstrated no difference in postoperative outcomes between patients with/without hypermobility (Beighton score >4) and/or knee hyperextension; in addition, Beighton scores did not correlate with postoperative symptoms, functional outcome scores, nor objective functional testing measures.[14] Because hypermobility is often combined with other API risk factors, these studies give insight into the problem but are underpowered to answer conclusively.

A la carte approach to "simple" cases of patellar instability

In the absence of displaced osteochondral fracture or loose bodies, standard of care for first-time LPD continues to be conservative management.[15] However, surgical indications are evolving to include failed nonoperative treatment and/or those patients whose risk stratification place them at high risk for recurrent LPD.

Dejour and Walch,[4,16] along with the "Lyonnaise" team, developed the "menu à la carte" patellar surgical treatment approach for patellar instability, by individualizing each anatomic risk factor present and surgically correcting it. More recently, the list of API risk factors has expanded as well as the list of surgical options, in particular, the addition of MPFL reconstruction. The cornerstone of patient evaluation continues to be detailing all risk factors contributing to recurrent LPD. However, it is not known *when* these factors have to be surgically corrected, and *at what numerical threshold,* for best outcomes. Specific surgical indications are discussed at length in sections of this issue pertaining to each of these risk factors, and the "menu options" to address each anatomic risk factor are summarized in **Table 1**.

The basic algorithmic approach for individuals with simple anatomic risk factors is summarized in **Fig. 1**. This à la carte approach offers a relatively straightforward methodology to addressing a singular risk factor for recurrence, but prioritization of risk factors and their indicated procedures is not described in such binary algorithms.

MULTIPLE RISK FACTORS AND COMPLEX SCENARIOS: REVISITING THE MENU FOR PATELLAR INSTABILITY

Current literature supports that additive risk factors result in additive risk for recurrent LPD (**Table 2**). The increased risk seems to be similar regardless of which specific combination of factors is present, suggesting that the number of risk factors is an independent variable that is important regardless of the specific risk factors. However, young age, in particular, open growth plates, is present in all models of additive risk for recurrence.

Risk factors for Lewallen and colleagues include the following: patella alta, trochlear dysplasia, chronologic age less than 25.

Risk factors for Arendt and colleagues include the following: open growth plates, sulcus angle greater than 154°, Insall-Salvati index greater than 1.3.

Risk factors for Jaquith and Parikh include the following: trochlear dysplasia, past contralateral history, skeletal immaturity, Caton-Deschamps index greater than 1.45.

Although existing literature clearly demonstrates that patients with multiple risk factors have an incremental risk for recurrent LPD, the interplay of these risk factors in surgical decision making is not straightforward. Many questions remain regarding how to best address these complex scenarios surgically. How does one weigh risk factors and their associated surgical procedures to optimize results and minimize

Table 1 Anatomic risk factors and their associated surgical procedures	
Risk Factor	**Surgical Procedures**
Trochlear dysplasia	Trochleoplasty Grooveplasty ("bumpectomy") Deepening trochleoplasty Recession wedge trochleoplasty
Patella alta	TTO with distalization Patellar tendon imbrication
Increased quadriceps vector	TTO with medialization Modified Grammont procedure Roux-Goldthwait procedure
Genu valgum	Varus distal femoral osteotomy (more common) Varus high tibial osteotomy
Rotational deformity (femoral or tibial)	Derotational distal femoral osteotomy Derotational tibial osteotomy

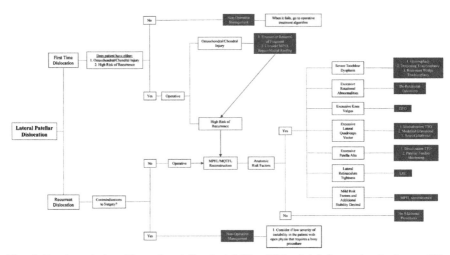

Fig. 1. Treatment algorithm of patellar instability. DFO, distal femoral osteotomy; LRL, lateral retinaculum lengthening; MPTL, medial patellotibial ligament; MQTFL, medial quadriceps tendon femoral ligament. (*Courtesy of* Betina Hinckel, MD, Royal Oak, MI.)

surgical morbidity and potential complications? Can addressing 1 risk factor mitigate the need to address others? Herein lies the need to take a deeper dive into the à la carte "menu" options, which the authors aim to do by discussing several specific and common scenarios.

Multiple and Combined Factors

Trochlear dysplasia is the most common risk factor for LPD and frequently coexists with PF malalignment.[5,6,8,17,18] Both trochlear dysplasia and malalignment influence patellar tracking, so the intricate relationship between them needs to be well understood. In those instances, one can choose to correct all factors, which increases morbidity, or one can correct the most relevant/severe factor in a manner to compensate for the other factors. Although patellar maltracking can be easily recognized on the physical examination, it is sometimes difficult to determine which anatomic factor

Table 2
Summary of studies reporting risk of recurrence with multiple concurrent risk factors

Number of Risk Factors	Risk of Recurrence (%)				
	0	1	2	3	4
Arendt, 2018[12]	7.7	22.7	50.9	78.5	—
Jaquith and Parikh,[10] 2017	13.8	30.1	53.6	74.8	88.4
Lewallen et al,[11] 2013	8.6	11.1–26.6*	29.6–60.2*	70.4	—

Risk factors for Lewallen et al include the following: patella alta, trochlear dysplasia, chronologic age less than 25.
  Risk factors for Arendt et al include the following: open growth plates, sulcus angle greater than 154°, Insall-Salvati index greater than 1.3.
  Risk factors for Jaquith and Parikh include the following: trochlear dysplasia, past contralateral history, skeletal immaturity, Caton-Deschamps index greater than 1.45.
  *Value range dependent on which risk factor was reported.

is predominantly responsible for the maltracking. In such instances, correlating physical examination tests and imaging measurements may be helpful. On the physical examination, a glide J-sign is more suggestive of bony malalignment (increased quadriceps vector and/or patella alta) combined with soft tissue issues (insufficiency of the medial stabilizers and/or tightness of the lateral retinaculum), whereas a clunk J-sign is more associated with severe dysplasia and a large trochlear bump.[19] Subluxation in extension suggests an increased quadriceps vector and/or patella alta. An increased lateral glide with (+) apprehension in deeper degrees of knee flexion indicates the presence of patella alta or a trochlear dysplasia that extends more distally and/or is more severe. On imaging studies, a trochlear bump/boss height of greater than 5 mm on lateral radiographs or greater than 8 mm on sagittal MRI views is considered significant (**Fig. 2**).[20]

Patella Alta and Increased Lateral Quadriceps Vector

Although increased lateral quadriceps vector was part of the original menu, many debate its value as an individual risk factor that needs correction in isolation[21,22]; it may play a greater role when combined with high grade trochlear dysplasia.[23]

Medial tibial tubercle transfer is often combined with distal transfer for treating patella alta or when combined with anteriorization to unload inferior/lateral patellar chondrosis. Having 2 indications for tibial tuberosity osteotomy (TTO), versus one, increases the benefit of performing it without further increasing the risk.

Trochlear Dysplasia and Patella Alta

The abnormalities of a dysplastic trochlea are more accentuated in the proximal trochlea. Thus, in some instances, the proximal dysplastic trochlea can be "bypassed"

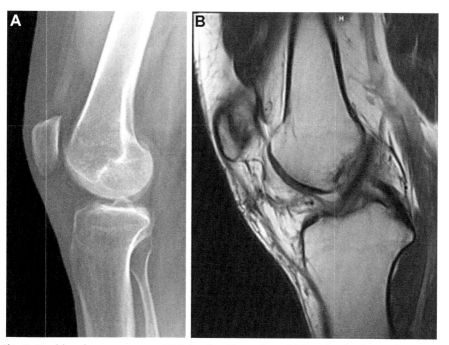

Fig. 2. Trochlear boss as seen on (A) lateral radiograph and (B) midsagittal cut of MRI in a patient with significant trochlear dysplasia without patella alta.

by distalizing the patella with a TTO. The ability to do so will depend on how far distal the trochlear dysplasia extends; otherwise stated, how short or long the trochlea is, and at what level it deepens. Typically, the more severe the trochlear dysplasia, the more prominent is its boss or anterior projection, limiting the utility of distal TTO as a preferred option (see **Fig. 2**). Therefore, this approach is more likely appropriate to the mildly dysplastic trochlea with a smaller trochlear spur and concurrent patella alta.

Trochlear Dysplasia and Large Quadriceps Vector

High-grade trochlear dysplasia (Dejour types B, C, and D) presents with a medialized trochlear groove, increasing the quadriceps vector[24] (**Fig. 3**).

The quadriceps vector can also be increased by knee valgus, rotational malalignment (increased femoral anteversion and increased knee rotation), and/or a lateralized patellar tendon insertion.[25–27] Understanding the components of a large quadriceps vector, as measured by the TT-TG, and correcting it at its source help to inform the preferred surgical technique, be it a trochleoplasty or a realignment procedure (eg, TTO medialization, distal femoral varus osteotomy, or femoral derotational osteotomy). An elevated TT-PCL has been used to help distinguish whether the elevated TT-TG is due to a lateralized tibial tubercle, or a more proximal abnormality (eg, knee valgus, knee rotation and/or femur torsion, or high-grade trochlear dysplasia). All these procedures have been shown to improve patellar tracking and patient-reported outcomes as well as decrease re-dislocation rates.[28–31] The correction of the more severe abnormality can compensate for lesser abnormalities and might be sufficient to improve patellar tracking. Many times, however, it is difficult to determine which is the more severe factor that is playing the major role in promoting instability. In general, trochlear dysplasia is more commonly the most relevant factor associated with PF instability, whereas malalignment is more frequently associated with anterior knee pain with/without patellar instability.[32] Therefore, trochleoplasty is primarily performed when treating patients with PF instability; on the other hand, rotational abnormalities of the lower extremity are much less often treated in the setting of PF instability, whereas more commonly corrected when treating PF pain.[33,34]

Another explanation for undertreatment of rotational issues may be an underrecognition or unfamiliarity with long bone rotational assessment, in addition to a wide

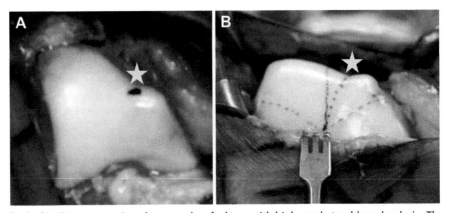

Fig. 3. (*A, B*) Intraoperative photographs of a knee with high-grade trochlear dysplasia. The sulcus (⭐) is relatively medialized due to the elevation of the central trochlea, thereby increasing the TT-TG by increasing the proximal measurement.

variation of reported "normal" anatomy leading to difficulty in identifying what constitutes "excessive" bony rotation.[35] However, increased limb version, in particular, increased femoral anteversion, is an evolving risk factor for LPD.[5,36,37] A recent study demonstrated that the treatment of patellar instability with increased femoral anteversion using MPFL reconstruction with derotational distal femoral osteotomy (DDFO) yields more favorable subjective and objective outcomes than MPFL reconstruction without DDFO, and this circumstance is more remarkable when the patients present with a preoperative high-grade J-sign.[34] In addition, unaddressed excessive femoral anteversion (>30°) combined with a J-sign is associated with greater patellar laxity, more residual J-signs, and poorer functional outcome scores even after TTO and MPFL reconstruction.[38] These findings suggest that TTO is not able to compensate for significant rotational abnormalities.

Regarding coronal plane alignment, debate continues on whether uncorrected tibiofemoral valgus places a patient at increased risk of re-dislocation or recurrent LPD, and if yes, at what threshold. Recent small series report favorable outcomes with valgus correction with and without medial soft tissue reconstruction.[39] Most investigators agree that when recurrent LPD is combined with at-risk lateral compartment cartilage (arthrosis, OCD), then a distal femoral osteotomy can be included in surgical patellar stabilization.[40]

Skeletal Immaturity and Bony Malalignment

The challenge in addressing skeletally immature patients with bony malalignment is 2-fold: the potential for changes in anatomy with continued skeletal growth, and the inability to use some "menu options," because of risk of physeal injury and resultant growth disturbance. On the other hand, continued longitudinal growth does introduce new "menu options" not available to adults, in the way of guided growth.

In skeletally immature patients, understanding how the anatomic risk factors for recurrent patellar instability change with age is important in determining when bony correction may be necessary. These changes are summarized in **Table 3**.

Femoral anteversion decreases by an average of 1.5° per year until reaching skeletal maturity, with average adult femoral anteversion of 12° to 15°.[41,42] Similarly, external tibial torsion results in a lateralized force vector on the patella. External tibial torsion increases dramatically in the first 5 to 7 years of life, with very minimal increases between 7 years of age and skeletal maturity.[43] Although diaphyseal derotational osteotomies of the femur and tibia can safely be performed in skeletally immature patients, consideration should be given to their respective bony alignment changes with age. Guided growth for correcting rotational malalignment has been studied in animal models but is not yet a treatment option in clinical practice; further studies are needed on that topic.[48]

Coronal alignment throughout skeletal development begins with significant genu varum in infants less than 1 year old, followed by marked genu valgum up to age 3 years, which subsequently decreases to approximate adult alignment (average 5°–6° valgus) by age 7 years.[44] Although adult-style metaphyseal osteotomies of the proximal tibia and distal femur for correction of genu valgum are not feasible in skeletally immature patients because of the risk of physeal injury, guided growth or hemiepiphysiodesis is a good option in patients with enough remaining expected growth. By selectively arresting growth of the medial distal femur with or without the medial proximal tibia, excessive genu valgum can be gradually corrected over the child's remaining period of growth, reducing the lateralized vector on the patella. This is generally indicated for skeletally immature patients with recurrent patellar instability and significant genu valgum greater than 10°, a mechanical lateral distal femoral angle less than 84°, and mechanical limb axis deviation outside of the lateral

Table 3
Expected change in anatomic risk factors in the skeletally immature individual

Anatomic Risk Factor	Change with Age
Femoral anteversion	Decrease[41,42]
Tibial torsion	Increase up to age 5–7 y; Minimal increase after 7 y[43]
Genu valgum	Increase age 1–3 y Decrease age 3–7 y Stable after 7 y[44]
Patella alta	Decrease[45]
Lateral quadriceps vector (measured by TT-TG)	Increase[46]
Trochlear dysplasia	Stable dysplasia severity (sulcus angle, Dejour classification); increased trochlear boss[47]

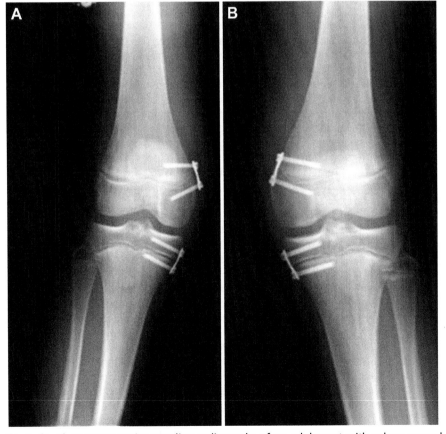

Fig. 4. (A, B) Anteroposterior standing radiographs of an adolescent with valgus coronal plane alignment, treated with hemiepiphysiodesis on the medial proximal tibia and medial distal femur. (Images courtesy of Elizabeth A. Arendt, MD.)

tibiofemoral compartment.[49] Hemiepiphysiodesis has proven effective at decreasing genu valgum and can be safely combined with MPFL reconstruction[49–51] (**Fig. 4**).

In the case of patellar instability with significantly increased lateral quadriceps vector or patella alta, traditionally a TTO (medializing or distalizing, respectively) is performed in conjunction with MPFL reconstruction to reduce risk of recurrent LPD. TTO cannot be performed, however, until after the tibial tubercle apophysis fuses to the tibial epiphysis between 14 and 18 years of age.[52] Patella alta has been found to decrease with age, closely approximating the average adult patellar height by age 10 years in female and 12 years in male patients.[45] In patients whose apophyses have not yet fused, patellar tendon imbrication is an effective means of correcting significant patella alta, with maintenance of correction seen at 2 years of follow-up.[53] Conversely, TT-TG distance increases with age.[46] There are many described soft tissue procedures aimed at medializing the distal pull on the patella, the most commonly cited being the Galeazzi tenodesis, the modified Grammont procedure, and the Roux-Goldthwait procedure. The indications for these historical procedures remain poorly defined, but they can be considered in the face of significantly elevated TT-TG and recurrent LPD in a skeletally immature individual.

Severity of trochlear dysplasia as indicated by sulcus angle and Dejour classification remains stable with skeletal growth, although the size of the trochlear boss seen in association with severe dysplasia increases with age.[47] Trochleoplasty is not an option for young patellar instability patients because of the risk for injury to the anterior extent of the distal femoral physis, which can result in a distal femur deformities from physeal arrest or hypergrowth. However, it may be safe for patients with minimal (less than 2 years) growth remaining.[54] Fortunately, for those who cannot undergo trochleoplasty, there is some evidence to suggest that in the absence of other risk factors (elevated TT-TG or patella alta), an isolated MPFL reconstruction is often sufficient.[55] In addition, early stabilization with MPFL reconstruction before physeal closure has been shown to have the potential to improve the femoral trochlear morphology.[56]

SUMMARY

PF instability is a multifactorial problem, and frequently patients have multiple anatomic risk factors present in their imaging profile.[1,8,9,12] Several studies have documented that a main factor in surgical failures is lack of acknowledgment or disregard of correctable anatomic risk factors.[57–59] Patella surgical stabilization has its roots in the "Lyonnaise" menu à la carte approach, which advocated surgical correction for each anatomic risk factor above a certain threshold. With the recognition of additional anatomic risk factors, and the routine use of advanced imaging to more objectively identify and document these risk factors, the practice of correcting all risk factors has morphed into a more individualized approach to the patient, with risk factors being weighed on a continuum of severity rather than having an absolute numerical threshold for anatomic values.

Despite this movement away from a dichotomous approach, clinical "best practice" mandates recognition of all risk factors, allowing for the surgical decision to include consideration of these risk factors. Only then can a surgical decision on which risk factor or factors to correct be made. To follow the teachings of the original "menu" by correcting all factors can be surgically challenging with additive risk to a successful outcome. Evidence-based studies are insufficiently powered at this time to be didactic when weighing multiple risk factors. This is due to the advancement in imaging that has increased variance across repetitive reads, and evolving data on "fringe" risk variables, for example, axial/coronal plane alignment. Many variables are continuous, not dichotomous, increasing the challenge to determine surgical thresholds and the number of variables potentially present in each individual.

Careful consideration of all contributing risk factors is necessary to identify and document. Blending physical examination findings with imaging measurements may be useful to help weigh the importance of individual risk factors. Referencing the menu à la carte options while prioritizing correction of multiple anatomic risk factors to create a surgical plan is challenging but a mandatory process in providing appropriate management of the patient with increased complexity owing to multiple risk factors.

CLINICS CARE POINTS

- Blending physical examination findings with imaging measurements may be useful to help weigh the importance of individual risk factors.
- Mandatory workup of the patient with recurrent lateral patellar dislocation requires identification and documentation of all patellar instability risk factors.
- Evidence-based studies are insufficiently powered at this time to be dogmatic when weighing multiple risk factors in creating a surgical plan.
- Shared decision making on surgical options, individualizing the patients' activity goals and their individual anatomic risk factors, continues to be best practice when addressing surgical patellar stabilization.

DISCLOSURE

Drs C.C. Chambers, B. Hinckel, and M.I. McCarthy have no relevant financial or nonfinancial interests to disclose. Dr E.A. Arendt's disclosures: *American Journal of Sports Medicine*: Editorial Board; International Society of Arthroscopy, Knee Surgery, and Orthopaedic Sports Medicine: Board or committee member; Knee Surgery, Sports Traumatology, Arthroscopy; Editorial Board; Smith & Nephew: Paid consultant and educational speaker.

REFERENCES

1. Huntington LS, Webster KE, Devitt BM, et al. Factors associated with an increased risk of recurrence after a first-time patellar dislocation: a systematic review and meta-analysis. Am J Sports Med 2020;48(10):2552–62.
2. Sillanpää P, Mattila VM, Iivonen T, et al. Incidence and risk factors of acute traumatic primary patellar dislocation. Med Sci Sports Exerc 2008;40(4):606–11.
3. Nomura E, Inoue M, Kurimura M. Chondral and osteochondral injuries associated with acute patellar dislocation. Arthroscopy 2003;19(7):717–21.
4. Dejour H, Walch G, Nove-Josserand L, et al. Factors of patellar instability: an anatomic radiographic study. Knee Surg Sports Traumatol Arthrosc 1994;2(1):19–26.
5. Imhoff FB, Funke V, Muench LN, et al. The complexity of bony malalignment in patellofemoral disorders: femoral and tibial torsion, trochlear dysplasia, TT–TG distance, and frontal mechanical axis correlate with each other. Knee Surg Sports Traumatol Arthrosc 2019;28(3):897–904.
6. Steensen RN, Bentley JC, Trinh TQ, et al. The prevalence and combined prevalences of anatomic factors associated with recurrent patellar dislocation: a magnetic resonance imaging study. Am J Sports Med 2015;43(4):921–7.

7. Xu Z, Zhang H, Chen J, et al. Femoral anteversion is related to tibial tubercle-trochlear groove distance in patients with patellar dislocation. Arthroscopy 2019;36(4):1114–20.
8. Arendt EA, England K, Agel J, et al. An analysis of knee anatomic imaging factors associated with primary lateral patellar dislocations. Knee Surg Sports Traumatol Arthrosc 2017;25(10):3099–107.
9. Balcarek P, Oberthür S, Hopfensitz S, et al. Which patellae are likely to redislocate? Knee Surg Sports Traumatol Arthrosc 2014;22(10):2308–14.
10. Jaquith BP, Parikh SN. Predictors of recurrent patellar instability in children and adolescents after first-time dislocation. J Pediatr Orthopaedics 2017;37(7):484–90.
11. Lewallen LW, McIntosh AL, Dahm DL. Predictors of recurrent instability after acute patellofemoral dislocation in pediatric and adolescent patients. Am J Sports Med 2013;41(3):575–81.
12. Arendt EA, Askenberger M, Agel J, et al. Risk of redislocation after primary patellar dislocation: a clinical prediction model based on magnetic resonance imaging variables. Am J Sports Med 2018;46(14):3385–90.
13. Howells NR, Eldridge JD. Medial patellofemoral ligament reconstruction for patellar instability in patients with hypermobility: a case control study. J Bone Joint Surg Br 2012;94(12):1655–9.
14. Hiemstra LA, Kerslake S, Kupfer N, et al. Generalized joint hypermobility does not influence clinical outcomes following isolated MPFL reconstruction for patellofemoral instability. Knee Surg Sports Traumatol Arthrosc 2019;27(11):3660–7.
15. Fithian DC, Paxton EW, Stone ML, et al. Epidemiology and natural history of acute patellar dislocation. Am J Sports Med 2004;32(5):1114–21.
16. Walch G, Dejour H. [Radiology in femoro-patellar pathology]. Acta Orthop Belg 1989;55(3):371–80. La radiologie dans la pathologie fémoro-patellaire.
17. Askenberger M, Janarv PM, Finnbogason T, et al. Morphology and anatomic patellar instability risk factors in first-time traumatic lateral patellar dislocations: a prospective magnetic resonance imaging study in skeletally immature children. Am J Sports Med 2017;45(1):50–8.
18. Kohlitz T, Scheffler S, Jung T, et al. Prevalence and patterns of anatomical risk factors in patients after patellar dislocation: a case control study using MRI. Eur Radiol 2012. https://doi.org/10.1007/s00330-012-2696-7.
19. Hinckel BB, Baumann CA, Fulkerson J. Distal realignment of the patellofemoral joint. In: Laprade RF, Chahla J, editors. Evidence-based management of complex knee injuries restoring the anatomy to achieve best outcomes. Amsterdam: Elsevier; 2020. p. 321–35. Chapter 28.
20. Pfirrmann CW, Zanetti M, Romero J, et al. Femoral trochlear dysplasia: MR findings. Radiology 2000;216(3):858–64.
21. Wagner D, Pfalzer F, Hingelbaum S, et al. The influence of risk factors on clinical outcomes following anatomical medial patellofemoral ligament (MPFL) reconstruction using the gracilis tendon. Knee Surg Sports Traumatol Arthrosc 2013;21(2):318–24.
22. Matsushita T, Kuroda R, Oka S, et al. Clinical outcomes of medial patellofemoral ligament reconstruction in patients with an increased tibial tuberosity-trochlear groove distance. Knee Surg Sports Traumatol Arthrosc 2014;22(10):2438–44.
23. Kita K, Tanaka Y, Toritsuka Y, et al. Factors affecting the outcomes of double-bundle medial patellofemoral ligament reconstruction for recurrent patellar dislocations evaluated by multivariate analysis. Am J Sports Med 2015;43(12):2988–96.

24. Keshmiri A, Schottle P, Peter C. Trochlear dysplasia relates to medial femoral condyle hypoplasia: an MRI-based study. Arch orthopaedic Trauma Surg 2019. https://doi.org/10.1007/s00402-019-03233-4.

25. Tensho K, Akaoka Y, Shimodaira H, et al. What components comprise the measurement of the tibial tuberosity-trochlear groove distance in a patellar dislocation population? J Bone Joint Surg Am 2015;97(17):1441–8.

26. Barahona M, Guzman M, Barrientos C, et al. The distance between tibial tubercle and trochlear groove correlates with knee articular torsion. J knee Surg 2020. https://doi.org/10.1055/s-0039-3402077.

27. Seitlinger G, Scheurecker G, Hogler R, et al. Tibial tubercle-posterior cruciate ligament distance: a new measurement to define the position of the tibial tubercle in patients with patellar dislocation. Evaluation Studies. Am J Sports Med 2012; 40(5):1119–25.

28. Longo UG, Vincenzo C, Mannering N, et al. Trochleoplasty techniques provide good clinical results in patients with trochlear dysplasia. Knee Surg Sports Traumatol Arthrosc 2017. https://doi.org/10.1007/s00167-017-4584-9.

29. Chen H, Zhao D, Xie J, et al. The outcomes of the modified Fulkerson osteotomy procedure to treat habitual patellar dislocation associated with high-grade trochlear dysplasia. BMC Musculoskelet Disord 2017;18(1):73.

30. Yang GM, Wang YY, Zuo LX, et al. Good outcomes of combined femoral derotation osteotomy and medial retinaculum plasty in patients with recurrent patellar dislocation. Orthop Surg 2019;11(4):578–85.

31. Wilson PL, Black SR, Ellis HB, et al. Distal femoral valgus and recurrent traumatic patellar instability: is an isolated varus producing distal femoral osteotomy a treatment option? J Pediatr orthopedics 2018;38(3):e162–7.

32. Balcarek P, Radebold T, Schulz X, et al. Geometry of torsional malalignment syndrome: trochlear dysplasia but not torsion predicts lateral patellar instability. Orthop J Sports Med 2019;7(3). 2325967119829790.

33. Stambough JB, Davis L, Szymanski DA, et al. Knee pain and activity outcomes after femoral derotation osteotomy for excessive femoral anteversion. J Pediatr Orthop 2018;38(10):503–9.

34. Zhang Z, Song G, Li Y, et al. Medial patellofemoral ligament reconstruction with or without derotational distal femoral osteotomy in treating recurrent patellar dislocation with increased femoral anteversion: a retrospective comparative study. Am J Sports Med 2021;49(1):200–6.

35. Shih YC, Chau MM, Arendt EA, et al. Measuring lower extremity rotational alignment: a review of methods and case studies of clinical applications. J Bone Joint Surg Am 2020;102(4):343–56.

36. Franciozi CE, Ambra LF, Albertoni LJ, et al. Increased femoral anteversion influence over surgically treated recurrent patellar instability patients. Arthroscopy 2017;33(3):633–40.

37. Kaiser P, Schmoelz W, Schoettle P, et al. Increased internal femoral torsion can be regarded as a risk factor for patellar instability - a biomechanical study. Clin Biomech (Bristol, Avon) 2017;47:103–9.

38. Zhang Z, Zhang H, Song G, et al. Increased femoral anteversion is associated with inferior clinical outcomes after MPFL reconstruction and combined tibial tubercle osteotomy for the treatment of recurrent patellar instability. Knee Surg Sports Traumatol Arthrosc 2020;28(7):2261–9.

39. Tan SHS, Hui SJ, Doshi C, et al. The outcomes of distal femoral varus osteotomy in patellofemoral instability: a systematic review and meta-analysis. J Knee Surg 2020;33(5):504–12.

40. Chahla J, Mitchell JJ, Liechti DJ, et al. Opening- and closing-wedge distal femoral osteotomy: a systematic review of outcomes for isolated lateral compartment osteoarthritis. Orthop J Sports Med 2016;4(6). 2325967116649901.
41. Svenningsen S, Apalset K, Terjesen T, et al. Regression of femoral anteversion. A prospective study of intoeing children. Acta Orthop Scand 1989;60(2):170–3.
42. Tönnis D, Heinecke A. Diminished femoral antetorsion syndrome: a cause of pain and osteoarthritis. J Pediatr Orthop 1991;11(4):419–31.
43. Kristiansen LP, Gunderson RB, Steen H, et al. The normal development of tibial torsion. Skeletal Radiol 2001;30(9):519–22.
44. Salenius P, Vankka E. The development of the tibiofemoral angle in children. J Bone Joint Surg Am 1975;57(2):259–61.
45. Walker P, Harris I, Leicester A. Patellar tendon-to-patella ratio in children. J Pediatr Orthop 1998;18(1):129–31.
46. Dickens AJ, Morrell NT, Doering A, et al. Tibial tubercle-trochlear groove distance: defining normal in a pediatric population. J Bone Joint Surg Am 2014; 96(4):318–24.
47. Parikh SN, Rajdev N, Sun Q. The growth of trochlear dysplasia during adolescence. J Pediatr Orthop 2018;38(6):e318–24.
48. Arami A, Bar-On E, Herman A, et al. Guiding femoral rotational growth in an animal model. J Bone Joint Surg Am 2013;95(22):2022–7.
49. Shah A, Parikh SN. Medial patellofemoral ligament reconstruction with growth modulation in children with patellar instability and genu valgum. Arthrosc Tech 2020;9(4):e565–74.
50. Kearney SP, Mosca VS. Selective hemiepiphyseodesis for patellar instability with associated genu valgum. J Orthop 2015;12(1):17–22.
51. Parikh SN, Redman C, Gopinathan NR. Simultaneous treatment for patellar instability and genu valgum in skeletally immature patients: a preliminary study. J Pediatr Orthop B 2019;28(2):132–8.
52. Beaty JKJ. Rockwood and Wilkins' fractures in children. 6th edition. Philadelphia: Lippincott Williams & Wilkins; 2005.
53. Patel RM, Gombosh M, Polster J, et al. Patellar tendon imbrication is a safe and efficacious technique to shorten the patellar tendon in patients with patella alta. Orthop J Sports Med 2020;8(10). 2325967120959318.
54. Nelitz M, Dreyhaupt J, Williams SRM. No growth disturbance after trochleoplasty for recurrent patellar dislocation in adolescents with open growth plates. Am J Sports Med 2018;46(13):3209–16.
55. Liu JN, Brady JM, Kalbian IL, et al. Clinical outcomes after isolated medial patellofemoral ligament reconstruction for patellar instability among patients with trochlear dysplasia. Am J Sports Med 2018;46(4):883–9.
56. Fu K, Duan G, Liu C, et al. Changes in femoral trochlear morphology following surgical correction of recurrent patellar dislocation associated with trochlear dysplasia in children. Bone Joint J 2018;100-b(6):811–21.
57. Chatterton A, Nielsen TG, Sørensen OG, et al. Clinical outcomes after revision surgery for medial patellofemoral ligament reconstruction. Knee Surg Sports Traumatol Arthrosc 2018;26(3):739–45.
58. Nelitz M, Williams RS, Lippacher S, et al. Analysis of failure and clinical outcome after unsuccessful medial patellofemoral ligament reconstruction in young patients. Int Orthop 2014;38(11):2265–72.
59. Feucht MJ, Mehl J, Forkel P, et al. Failure analysis in patients with patellar redislocation after primary isolated medial patellofemoral ligament reconstruction. Orthop J Sports Med 2020;8(6). 2325967120926178.

Fixed (Congenital) Patellar Dislocation

Phillip T. Grisdela, MD, Nikolaos Paschos, MD, PhD, Miho J. Tanaka, MD*

KEYWORDS

- Knee • Congenital patellar dislocation • Fixed patellar dislocation • Realignment
- Lateral release

KEY POINTS

- Congenital dislocation of the patella is a fixed, lateral dislocation of the patella that is not reducible without surgical correction.
- Diagnosis of congenital dislocation of the patella is frequently delayed, and must be suspected among patients with delayed ambulation, genu valgum, external tibial rotation, and flexion contracture of the knee.
- Surgical treatment techniques vary, but consist of lateral release, medial soft tissue stabilization, quadriceps lengthening, and distal realignment.

INTRODUCTION

Congenital dislocation of the patella (CDP) is a rare condition of unknown incidence that is marked by a fixed dislocation of the patella on the lateral border of the femoral condyle and is unable to be reduced without surgery. The first description of a congenital dislocation was by Singer in 1856, and the first surgical treatment was by Goldthwait in 1869.[1,2] Conn defined the condition in 1925 as having 4 requirements: (1) a permanent lateral patellar dislocation, (2) inability of the patient to actively extend the knee, (3) preservation of passive knee range of motion, and (4) absence of the patella from the trochlea since birth.[3,4]

Some investigators view CDP as a part of a larger spectrum of disease, including developmental dysplasia of the patellofemoral joint that can lead to a fixed patellar dislocation years after birth.[5] Additionally, habitual, or "obligatory" dislocation of the patella, in which the patella dislocates and relocates involuntarily as the knee moves from flexion to extension, has been proposed as another manifestation of congenital dislocation if present at birth.[6] Obligatory dislocation typically develops at a later age and does not require surgery as frequently.[6,7] Because the disease exists on a

Department of Orthopaedic Surgery, Massachusetts General Hospital, Harvard Medical School, 55 Fruit Street, Boston, MA 02114, USA
* Corresponding author. 175 Cambridge Street, Suite 400, Boston, MA 02114.
E-mail address: Mtanaka5@mgh.harvard.edu

Clin Sports Med 41 (2022) 123–136
https://doi.org/10.1016/j.csm.2021.07.010
0278-5919/22/© 2021 Elsevier Inc. All rights reserved.

spectrum, the diagnosis of fixed patellar dislocation is frequently delayed. Additionally, evaluation and imaging of this condition can be limited by the fact that the fixed dislocated patella is frequently smaller and ossifies later than the usual 3 to 5 years of age.[8] This article reviews the etiology, pathophysiology, evaluation, and treatment of this unique condition along the spectrum of patellofemoral disease.

ETIOLOGY

Possible etiologies of fixed patellar dislocation include malrotation of the myotome involving the quadriceps and patella, which occurs in utero at the 8th to 9th weeks of gestation,[1] leading to persistent lateral position of the extensor mechanism. Fixed patellar dislocation has been associated with many congenital syndromes, which should be considered at the time of evaluation. Commonly associated syndromes and findings are presented in **Table 1**.[9–22] Additional rare causes include iatrogenic quadriceps fibrosis from repeated intramuscular injections of antibiotic causing progressive habitual dislocation leading to fixed dislocation of the patella.[23] Although CDP does not have a clear genetic association, some investigators have suggested that the condition is found more frequently bilaterally and may be inherited in an autosomal-dominant fashion.[24–26] Given these associations and the frequent delays in diagnosis, it is prudent to perform a thorough musculoskeletal examination of patients with these conditions, particularly those who present with the typical findings of genu valgus, flexion contracture, and external tibial rotation.

PATHOPHYSIOLOGY

A fixed patellar dislocation involves contraction of the lateral structures and elongation of the medial soft tissue structures. The patella lateralizes beyond the lateral femoral condyle and becomes entrapped anteriorly by the fascia lata, laterally by the iliotibial band, and posteriorly by the intermuscular septum.[27] Gao and colleagues[28] described 7 anatomic findings that are consistent with this condition: (1) contracture and fibrosis of mainly the vastus lateralis, which pulls the quadriceps musculature to the anterolateral aspect of the knee joint, (2) a contracted iliotibial band that is adhered to the patella and prevents reduction, (3) a globally contracted lateral joint capsule and lax medial joint capsule, (4) a loose and atrophic vastus medialis, (5) lateral insertion of the patellar tendon on the tibia, (6) an externally rotated tibia with valgus deformity at the knee, and (7) a hypoplastic, flattened patella with a shallow, empty trochlear groove. These findings were supported by a cadaveric study of a stillborn child with congenital patellar dislocation examined by Ghanem and colleagues.[29]

In the setting of a fixed lateral patellar dislocation, the extensor mechanism has dislocated posterior to the center of rotation of the knee. This dislocation causes the quadriceps muscles to act as paradoxic drivers of knee flexion rather than knee extension. Because of this, patients with fixed patellar dislocation typically have weakened quadriceps function and altered gait kinematics. Patients may be able to ambulate with a unilateral fixed dislocation by flexing the hip of the affected leg in the stance phase of the well leg, tensioning the posterior capsule and ligamentous structures of the knee, and pushing their body weight forward to advance. As patients age with worsening contracture, the tibia externally rotates and they can ambulate with stability from collateral ligaments and flexion of the adductor musculature.[27]

Table 1
Associated conditions with congenital patellar dislocation, their inheritance patterns, diagnostic findings, and other characteristics

Syndrome	Genetic Inheritance	Diagnostic Findings	Other Characteristics
Down syndrome	Trisomy 21	Joint hyperlaxity and hypotonia of the musculature	Atlantoaxial and atlanto-occipital instability, cardiac abnormalities, scoliosis, pes planus, slipped capital femoral epiphysis, hip instability
Larsen's syndrome	Autosomal dominant and recessive reported	Hyperelasticity of the joints with associated knee, hip and elbow dislocations	Hypertelorism, equinovarus feet, supernumerary ossification of the hands and feet, short stature and cardiac disease
Thrombocytopenia absent radius	Both autosomal recessive and autosomal dominant reported	Platelets <5K, absent radius, thumbs present	Short stature, macrocephaly, septal defects, lactose intolerance
Williams Beuren syndrome	Chromosome 7 deletion, Autosomal dominant	Hyperelasticity owing to altered elastin function	Aortic stenosis, short stature, "elfin facies," hypercalcemia, intellectual delay
Nail patella syndrome	Autosomal dominant	Hypoplastic/absent patella	Fingernail dysplasia, hypoplasia of the radial head and capitellum, "iliac horns," frequent renal involvement
Fibular hemimelia	Variable	Tibial procurvatum, partial to completely absent fibula, anterior cruciate ligament and posterior cruciate ligament deficiency common	Talipes equinovarus, tarsal coalition, upper extremity abnormalities, cardiac and renal abnormalities, femoral shortening, acetabular dysplasia
Kabuki syndrome	Variable	Arched/broad eyebrows, short columella with depressed nasal tip, large prominent/cupped ears, persistent fingertip pads	Ligamentous laxity, joint dislocation, intellectual delay, cardiac/renal abnormalities, failure to thrive, hypotonia

(continued on next page)

Table 1 (continued)			
Syndrome	Genetic Inheritance	Diagnostic Findings	Other Characteristics
Foot abnormalities (vertical talus, talipes equinovarus)	Slight male predominance	Evaluate for concomitant knee pathology in cases of delayed ambulation	Club foot will be cavus, forefoot adducted, varus and equinus; vertical talus will have rocker-bottom foot with equinovalgus deformity
Ellis Van–Creveld syndrome	Autosomal recessive	Significant genu valgum deformity, "saucer-like" depression of lateral tibial plateau	Associated with eastern Pennsylvania Amish, short stature, polydactyly, cardiac anomalies, dysplastic fingernails and teeth

EVALUATION

History

In many cases, the initial presentation of congenital patellar dislocation is associated with delayed ambulation. Caretakers may also report deformities or abnormalities in gait or range of motion. A thorough history should be obtained to elicit the timing of onset to assess the contribution of traumatic or developmental conditions. Comprehensive history taking should be performed to identify any associated syndromes based on a thorough discussion of medical history and symptoms, as well as a family history of genetic disorders.

Examination

The primary goal of the examination is to identify the contributors to the patient's functional deficits, including malalignment, flexion contracture, lateral contracture, joint stability, and strength. In patients who are ambulatory, gait should be evaluated carefully for compensatory changes that include contralateral hip flexion, as well as external rotation of the affected leg with engagement of the adductor muscles.[27]

Standing or supine evaluation of alignment should include assessment for genu valgus. External tibial rotation can be assessed with the patient prone, with a foot axis of more than 10° from the thigh axis indicating abnormal rotational alignment (**Fig. 1**).[30] Frontal plane alignment can also identify a lateralized tibial tuberosity, which can be quantified by the Q angle.

Range of motion should be assessed actively and passively, with careful differentiation between functional limitation from the patella dislocation versus that from muscle contracture. The extremities should be evaluated for quadriceps, hamstring, and abductor contractures. Particular attention should be paid to the degree of knee flexion attainable if the patella is able to be held in a reduced position, because this can indicate shortening of the extensor mechanism. Vastus lateralis contracture and

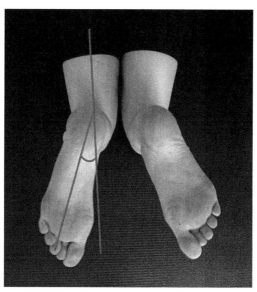

Fig. 1. Thigh–foot angle is determined to assess for tibial external rotation by measuring the angle between the thigh and the axis of the hindfoot/tibia with the patient in a prone position.

contracture of the iliotibial band can be assessed using Ober's test. The quadriceps muscle group is evaluated for atrophy, particularly in the vastus medialis. Strength testing is performed to identify abnormalities in the quadriceps, hamstring, adductor, and abductor muscle groups.

A detailed examination of the patellofemoral joint includes identification of the location, morphology, and mobility of the patella. A careful assessment should consider the abnormal size and position of the patella that may complicate the examination. Because the patella is generally fixed and dislocated laterally, an empty trochlea may be palpated. The knee is taken through range of motion to assess for changes in patellar position or stability. A medially directed force can be applied to the patella to determine the severity of lateral contracture and whether the position of the patella can be partially or completely corrected at a given flexion angle.

In patients without a known or diagnosed syndrome, a focused examination to evaluate for findings associated with suspected genetic or congenital syndromes should take place. This process includes an evaluation for joint laxity in the knee and hip. Hands and feet can be evaluated for supernumerary ossification associated with Larsen's syndrome, and fingernails should be assessed for dysplasia consistent with nail patella syndrome. Elbows can be assessed for instability owing to hypoplasia of the radial head and capitellum, which can occur in nail patella syndrome. Abnormalities of the feet including vertical talus or talipes equinovarus may be identified (**Fig. 2**). Common conditions and their associated findings are reviewed in **Table 1**.

Imaging

Ultrasound examination

Ultrasound imaging is the primary mode for the evaluation of patients with congenital patellar dislocation before ossification of the patella. Ossification of the patella typically occurs at approximately 3 to 5 years of age, but may be delayed in cases of

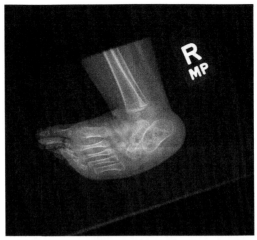

Fig. 2. Right foot radiograph demonstrates talipes equinovarus which can occur in some patients with congenital patellar dislocation.

congenital patellar dislocations.[6] Ultrasound evaluation can be used to assess the position and morphology of the unossified patella, as well as to evaluate the trochlea and the surrounding structures.

Radiographs

Radiographs of the knee are helpful in assessing congenital patellar dislocation after the age of 5 years, when ossification of the patella occurs (**Fig. 3**). Weightbearing anteroposterior views and standing long leg radiographs can assess for coronal plane abnormalities (**Fig. 4**). Axial and lateral views of the knee can provide information on the morphology and location of the patella, as well as the morphology of the trochlea, to determine the contributors of morphologic risk factors to patellar dislocation.

In cases where a congenital syndrome is not yet diagnosed, obtaining additional images of other extremities may aid in identifying the underlying diagnosis. Radiographs

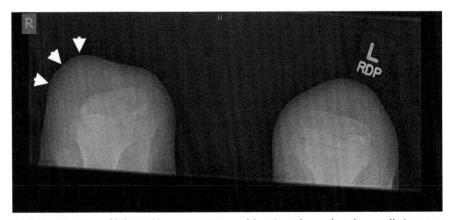

Fig. 3. Sunrise view of bilateral knees in a 4-year-old patient shows that the patella is not yet ossified. Silhouette of the patella (indicated by white arrows) demonstrates asymmetry with lateralization of the patella in the right knee.

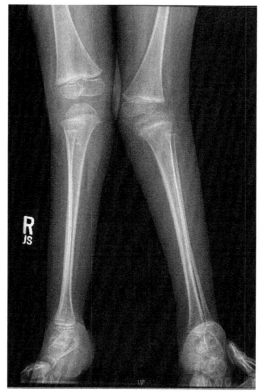

Fig. 4. Radiograph of the bilateral lower extremities demonstrates coronal plane valgus abnormality of the left knee in a skeletally immature patient.

of the hands may help identify abnormal ossification as found in Larsen's syndrome, and radiographs of the elbows may identify hypoplasia of the radial head or capitellum frequently associated with nail patella syndrome (**Fig. 5**).

MRI

MRI allows for an assessment of the soft tissue and cartilaginous morphology associated with this congenital patellar dislocation, with greater detail than in other modalities (**Fig. 6**). In addition to the position and morphology of the patella and trochlea, the integrity and quality of the surrounding soft tissue structures can be assessed. Axial images may show attenuation of the medial retinaculum or thickening of the lateral retinaculum. The use of MRI in the pediatric population may be limited by the need for anesthesia in children and this point should be taken into consideration after evaluating other, more accessible modalities. Computed tomography scan is typically avoided given the high radiation burden in this patient population, but can further demonstrate the morphology of the patellofemoral joint and surrounding bony structures (**Fig. 7**).[8,31]

TREATMENT
Nonoperative Management

Nonoperative management of a fixed patellar dislocation can be performed in the preoperative period; it typically does not serve as a definitive treatment, because the

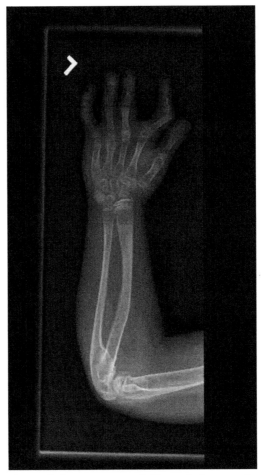

Fig. 5. Left elbow radiograph demonstrates radial hypoplasia, as can be seen in nail patella syndrome. (Image courtesy of F. Joseph Simeone, MD.)

condition by definition is irreducible by closed means. Serial casting or bracing can be a useful tool in the preoperative time period to improve flexion contracture.[32] Uncorrected, CDP can drive worsening flexion contracture, with compensatory external rotation of the tibia to allow for ambulation reliant on the collateral ligaments of the knee for support and the adductor musculature for propulsion.[27] The genu valgus deformity of the condition can drive early lateral compartment osteoarthritis of the affected knee.[33] However, there are reports of patients with missed CDP presenting well into adulthood, with 2 cases in the literature of a 16-year-old patient and a 51-year-old patient refusing surgical intervention for their fixed patellar dislocation because they did not experience significant functional deficit.[34,35]

Surgical Treatment

Many authors advocate for early surgical management before the onset of ambulation, although given the delays in diagnosis, some patients do not present until their adolescent or teen years, with some notable cases being identified in late adulthood.[32,36]

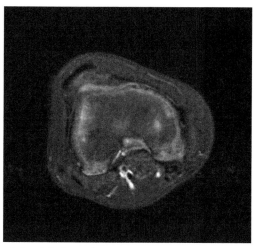

Fig. 6. T2 axial MRI of the right knee demonstrates a dysplastic trochlea with lateralization of a hypoplastic patella.

Surgical management focuses on restoring patellar position, stability, and the integrity of the extensor mechanism. Although multiple and varied surgical techniques have been described to address CDP, each of these commonly addresses the following abnormalities: (1) correction of coronal or rotational malalignment is performed with a distal realignment procedure; (2) release of the lateral tissues is performed to allow for centralization of the patella; (3) medial soft tissue stabilization with imbrication, advancement, or reconstruction is performed to limit lateral patellar translation; and (4) shortening of the extensor mechanism is addressed with quadriceps lengthening

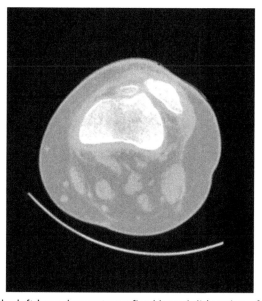

Fig. 7. CT scan of the left knee demonstrates fixed lateral dislocation of the patella.

and/or release. In addition, bony procedures to correct genu valgum or excessive tibial torsion (>45°) may be required, as well as the release of severe flexion contractures with posterior release or lengthening procedures.

Large series of procedures to address this uncommon condition have not been described. Goldthwaite described performing a lateral capsular release with reattachment of the patellar tendon to the sartorius attachment on one side and a tibial tubercle transfer on the contralateral side. Although a distal femoral osteotomy was undertaken bilaterally to improve knee range of motion, results were reported as satisfactory at the 2-year follow-up.[1,2] Conn and colleagues reported another method incorporating lateral release, medial capsular imbrication and lateral lengthening with graft from the medial capsule to close the lateral defect. Although the length of follow-up was not recorded, the authors reported the functional result as good.[1] Goldthwaite's original procedure has since been modified to the well-known Roux–Goldthwaite procedure, in which a lateral retinacular release, transfer of the lateral tibial insertion of the patellar tendon under the medial aspect, medial retinacular plication with vastus medialis oblique advancement is performed, which has been commonly used with good results in the treatment of recurrent patellar dislocations.[37]

Stanisavljevic and colleagues[1] described an extensive subperiosteal elevation of the vastus lateralis from 4 cm under the greater trochanter with excision of the fascia lata and division of the patellar tendon longitudinally with transfer of the lateral insertion under the medial tendon and sutured as medially as possible, combined with plication of medial structures and closure of the lateral defect with fascia lata harvested at the beginning of the surgery. The results with this procedure have generally been favorable, with Sever and colleagues[7] reporting on 12 patients with fixed and habitual dislocations, in which 11 patients had no redislocation at 46.2 months after undergoing the procedure at a mean age of 7 years. In contrast, Camathias and colleagues[38] reported 80% redislocation rates after 7.5 years for patients with habitual or congenital patellar dislocation; however, patients in their group underwent surgery at a mean of 12.8 years of age, and older age at the time of surgery has been associated with worse outcomes. Gordon and Schoenecker[39] modified the Stanisavljevic procedure with a patellar tendon transfer in skeletally immature patients and tibial tubercle transfer in skeletally mature patients, leaving the lateral defect open. In their series of 17 knees in 11 patients, all with fixed lateral dislocation who underwent surgery at a mean age of 7 years, the authors reported that all patients had a marked increase in activity tolerance and relief of pain at a follow-up period of 5.1 years, with average flexion contracture improved from 15° preoperatively to 2° postoperatively.[39]

Langenskiold and Ritsila[40] described a technique in which the iliotibial band and biceps femoris were divided obliquely, and a distal realignment was performed by releasing the patellar tendon distally from the tibial tubercle and reattaching to a socket in the tibial metaphysis distal to the growth plate. Langenskiold's original series in 12 patients had good reported outcomes at over 13 years of follow-up, with all but 2 of 12 patients obtaining full range of motion.[40] This procedure has been modified with either a "buckle" formed by passing the patellar tendon through a buttonhole of distal joint capsule as demonstrated by Paton and colleagues, or by keeping the patellar tendon extrasynovial as described by Paley and colleagues.[41,42] The Paley modification did report 1 episode of overmedialization in a patient with CDP that did not require surgical management and 2 redislocations in the same patient in a chronic patellar dislocation, but otherwise reported satisfaction in 8 of 13 patients.[42]

The 4-in-1 extensor realignment consists of an extensive lateral release, Roux-Goldthwait procedure, Galeazzi procedure to transfer the semitendinosus to the superolateral patella through a transosseous drill hole, and vastus medialis oblique advancement. In a series of fixed and habitual patellar dislocations, Danino and colleagues[43] reported on 6 knees with fixed dislocation, with a mean age of 8.6 ± 2.4 years and a follow-up of 53.5 months. In these knees, the authors reported 100% had returned to activities of daily living and sport at a duration of 20 weeks, with a mean Kujala score of 91.5. One of the 6 knees (17%) suffered repeat dislocation, and the authors noted that long-term bracing was more commonly needed (75% vs 17%) in fixed dislocations, when compared with habitual dislocators.[43] Finally, İnan and colleagues[44] reported on 14 knees treated with tensor fascia lata transfer behind the patellar tendon and under the semitendinosus tendon, before attachment on the medial patella, and combined with vastus lateralis resection, medial capsular plication and Z-plasty of the rectus femoris. At an average follow-up of 37.6 months, range of motion and genu valgum and recurvatum deformity improved in all patients, with 2 of the 9 patients having recurrent lateral subluxation requiring revision medial plication.[44]

The most common complication after surgical treatment for congenital patellar dislocation is persistent flexion contracture, as well as recurrent dislocation requiring revision surgery, with more recent studies reporting rates of 25% after treatment for CDP.[43,44] Additional reported complications have included superficial wound infections and a case of peroneal neuropraxia, which resolved without treatment.[39]

Missed or untreated fixed patellar dislocation is associated with worsening flexion contracture, external tibial rotation and valgus deformity, ultimately resulting in early onset osteoarthritis focused on the lateral compartment. This can be managed with medial closed-wedge osteotomy and soft tissue reconstruction and tibial tubercle transfer with use of hamstring tendon transfer as described by Yoshvin and colleagues[45] in a series of 5 patients at average age of 29.6 years, or by rotational osteotomies combined with tibial tuberosity transfer as described by Ramaswamy and colleagues.[46] Noda and colleagues[47] report on a staged procedure using an Ilizarov frame to correct valgus deformity and lengthen the affected limb before realignment. This issue has been addressed in adult patients with total knee arthroplasty both with and without reduction of the extensor mechanism, although many cases still had range of motion deficits postoperatively. Only 1 of the 10 cases included in this review reported full range of motion.[33,48–50] At the other end of the spectrum, there are reports of patients presenting as late as their 50s with fixed dislocation without significant functional deficit who continue to decline surgical intervention.[34,35] Owing to the uncommon nature of this condition as well as the numerous described treatment options, only small series of patients and reported outcomes currently exist. Further studies are needed to identify the optimal technique and indication for each component of the surgical management of congenital patellar dislocations.

SUMMARY

CDP is a rare condition that can be associated with multiple other congenital syndromes that consists of a fixed, lateral dislocation of the patella that is irreducible without surgical management. Fixed dislocation has been described on a spectrum that includes obligatory dislocation, which occurs with knee flexion and reduces with knee extension. Patients demonstrate flexion contracture, loss of active knee extension, and increased tibial external rotation. Treatment, by definition, requires surgical management to reduce the patella. Multiple procedures have been described, but, in general, management focuses on releasing the contracted lateral structures, medial soft tissue stabilization, quadriceps lengthening, and transfer of the patellar tendon or tibial tubercle depending on the skeletal maturity of the patient. Results in small series are generally favorable, with persistent flexion contracture and redisloca-tion as the most common complications reported. Further study is required of the eti-ology and ideal timing as well as treatment strategy for this uncommon condition.

CLINICS CARE POINTS

- CDP is a fixed, lateral dislocation of the patella that is not reducible without surgical correction.
- The diagnosis of CDP is frequently delayed, and must be suspected among patients with delayed ambulation, genu valgum, external tibial rotation, and flexion contracture of the knee.
- Surgical treatment techniques vary, but consist of lateral release, medial soft tissue stabilization, quadriceps lengthening, and distal realignment.

DISCLOSURE

The authors report that there are no commercial or financial conflicts of interest, there was no outside funding for this work.

REFERENCES

1. Stanisavljevic S, Zemenick G, Miller D. Congenital, irreducible, permanent lateral dislocation of the patella. Clin Orthop Relat Res 1976;116:190–9.
2. Goldthwait JEV. Permanent dislocation of the patella. The report of a case of twenty years' duration, successfully treated by transplantation of the patella ten-dons with the tubercle of the tibia. Ann Surg 1899;29(1):62–8.
3. Jones RD, Fisher RL, Curtis BH. Congenital dislocation of the patella. Clin Orthop Relat Res 1976;119:177–83.
4. Stern M. Persistent congenital dislocation of the patella. Report of a case. J Int Coll Surg 1964;41:654–6.
5. Paton RW, Kim WY, Bonshahi A. Non traumatic dislocation of the patella in chil-dren: the case for a dysplastic aetiology. Acta Orthop Belg 2005;71(4):435–8.
6. Eilert RE. Congenital dislocation of the patella. Clin Orthop Relat Res 2001; 389:22–9.
7. Sever R, Fishkin M, Hemo Y, et al. Surgical treatment of congenital and obligatory dislocation of the patella in children. J Pediatr Orthop 2019;39(8):436–40.
8. Koplewitz B, Babyn P, Cole W. Congenital dislocation of the patella. Am J Roent-gol 2005;8:200–4.
9. Ilyas G, Eren TK, Kaptan AY, et al. Bilateral congenital dislocation of the patella associated with synostosis of proximal tibiofibular and proximal radioulnar joints: a case report. Eklem Hastalik Cerrahisi 2018;29(2):123–7.
10. Wang CH, Shu L, Ma LF, et al. Medial and lateral retinaculum plasty for congenital patellar dislocation due to small patella syndrome. Orthopedics 2013;36(11): 1418–23.
11. Weiner DS, Tank JC, Jonah D, et al. An operative approach to address severe genu valgum deformity in the Ellis-van Creveld syndrome. J Child Orthop 2014; 8(1):61–9.
12. Kurosawa K, Kawame H, Ochiai Y, et al. Patellar dislocation in Kabuki syndrome. Am J Med Genet 2002;108(2):160–3.
13. Green A. The pediatric foot and ankle. Pediatr Clin North Am 2020;67(1):169–83.

14. Wilson M, Carter IB. Williams syndrome. StatPearls; 2021. Available at: http://www.ncbi.nlm.nih.gov/pubmed/31334998.
15. Bettuzzi C, Lampasi M, Magnani M, et al. Surgical treatment of patellar dislocation in children with down syndrome: a 3- to 11-year follow-up study. Knee Surg Sport Traumatol Arthrosc 2009;17(4):334–40.
16. Carpintero P, Mesa M, Carpintero A. Bilateral congenital dislocation of the patella. Acta Orthop Belg 1996;62(2):113–5.
17. Laville J, Lakermance P, Limouzy F. Larsen's syndrome: review of the literature and analysis of thirty-eight cases. J Pediatr Orthop 1994;14:63–73.
18. Marumo K, Fujii K, Tanaka T, et al. Surgical management of congenital permanent dislocation of the patella in nail patella syndrome by Stanisavljevic procedure. J Orthop Sci 1999;4(6):446–9.
19. Boniel S, Szymańska K, Śmigiel R, et al. Kabuki syndrome-clinical review with molecular aspects. Genes (Basel) 2021;12(4):468.
20. de Ybarrondo L, Barratt MS. Thrombocytopenia absent radius syndrome. Pediatr Rev 2011;32(9):399–400.
21. Hamdy RC, Makhdom AM, Saran N, et al. Congenital fibular deficiency. J Am Acad Orthop Surg 2014;22(4):246–55.
22. Muensterer OJ, Berdon W, McManus C, et al. Ellis–van Creveld syndrome: its history. Pediatr Radiol 2013;43(8):1030–6.
23. Hung NN, Tan D, Do Ngoc Hien N. Patellar dislocation due to iatrogenic quadriceps fibrosis: results of operative treatment in 54 cases. J Child Orthop 2014;8(1):49–59.
24. Robinson AHN, Aladin A, Green AJ, et al. Congenital dislocation of the patella - The genetics and conservative management. Knee 1998;5(3):235–7.
25. Mumford EB. Congenital dislocation of the patella; case report with history of four generations. J Bone Joint Surg Am 1947;29(4):1083–6.
26. Rosa JM, Carvalho AD, Coutinho LL, et al. Surgical treatment for congenital dislocation of the patella in a young adult: a case report. JBJS Case Connect 2019;9(4):1–6.
27. Zeier FG, Dissanayake C. Congenital dislocation of the patella. Clin Orthop Relat Res 1980;148:140–6.
28. Gao G, Lee E, Bose K. Surgical management of congenital and habitual dislocation of the patella. J Pediatr Orthop 1990;10(2):255–60.
29. Ghanem I, Wattincourt L, Seringe R. Congenital dislocation of the patella. Part I: pathologic anatomy. J Pediatr Orthop 2000;20(6):812–6.
30. Lincoln TL, Suen PW. Common rotational variations in children. J Am Acad Orthop Surg 2003;11(5):312–20.
31. Miguel Sá P, Raposo F, Santos Carvalho M, et al. Congenital dislocation of the patella – clinical case. Rev Bras Ortop (English Ed 2016;51(1):109–12.
32. Wada A, Fujii T, Takamura K, et al. Congenital dislocation of the patella. J Child Orthop 2008;2(2):119–23.
33. Dao Q, Chen DB, Scott RD. Proximal patellar quadricepsplasty realignment during total knee arthroplasty for irreducible congenital dislocation of the patella: a report of two cases. J Bone Joint Surg Am 2010;92(14):2457–61.
34. Bistolfi A, Massazza G, Backstein D, et al. Adult congenital permanent bilateral dislocation of the patella with full knee function: case report and literature review. Case Rep Med 2012;2012:182795.
35. Tokgöz MA, Çavuşoğlu AT, Ayanoğlu T, et al. Neglected bilateral congenital dislocation of the patella. Eklem Hastalik Cerrahisi 2017;28(2):128–31.

36. Ghanem I, Wattincourt L, Seringe R. Congenital dislocation of the patella. Part II: orthopaedic management. J Pediatr Orthop 2000;20(6):817–22.
37. Fondren FB, Goldner JL, Bassett FH. Recurrent dislocation of the patella treated by the modified Roux-Goldthwait procedure. A prospective study of forty-seven knees. J Bone Joint Surg Am 1985;67(7):993–1005.
38. Camathias C, Rutz E, Götze M, et al. Poor outcome at 7.5 years after Stanisavljevic quadriceps transposition for patello-femoral instability. Arch Orthop Trauma Surg 2014;134(4):473–8.
39. Gordon JE, Schoenecker PL. Surgical treatment of congenital dislocation of the patella. J Pediatr Orthop 1999;19(2):260–4.
40. Langenskiold A, Ritsila V. Congenital dislocation of the patella and its operative treatment. J Pediatr Orthop 1992;12:315–23.
41. Paton RW, Bonshahi AY, Kim WY. Congenital and irreducible non-traumatic dislocation of the patella - a modified soft tissue procedure. Knee 2004;11(2):117–20.
42. Ramos O, Burke C, Lewis M, et al. Modified langenskiöld procedure for chronic, recurrent, and congenital patellar dislocation. J Child Orthop 2020;14(4):318–29.
43. Danino B, Deliberato D, Abousamra O, et al. Four-in-one extensor realignment for the treatment of obligatory or fixed, lateral patellar instability in skeletally immature knee. J Pediatr Orthop 2020;40(9):503–8.
44. İnan M, Sarıkaya İA, Şeker A, et al. A combined procedure for irreducible dislocation of patella in children with ligamentous laxity: a preliminary report. Acta Orthop Traumatol Turc 2015;49(5):530–8.
45. Yoshvin S, Southern EP, Wang Y. Surgical treatment of congenital patellar dislocation in skeletally mature patients: surgical technique and case series. Eur J Orthop Surg Traumatol 2015;25(6):1081–6.
46. Ramaswamy R, Kosashvili Y, Murnaghan JJ, et al. Bilateral rotational osteotomies of the proximal tibiae and tibial tuberosity distal transfers for the treatment of congenital lateral dislocations of patellae: a case report and literature review. Knee 2009;16(6):507–11.
47. Noda M, Saegusa Y, Kashiwagi N, et al. Surgical treatment for permanent dislocation of the patella in adults. Orthopedics 2011;34(12):948–51.
48. Yamanaka H, Kawamoto T, Tamai H, et al. Total knee arthroplasty in a patient with bilateral congenital dislocation of the patella treated with a different method in each knee. Case Rep Orthop 2015;2015:890315.
49. Bergquist PE, Baumann PA, Finn HA. Total knee arthroplasty in an adult with congenital dislocation of the patella. J Arthroplasty 2001;16(3):384–8.
50. Kumagi M, Ikeda S, Uchida K, et al. Total knee replacement for osteoarthritis of the knee with congenital dislocation of the patella. J Bone Joint Surg Br 2007; 89(11):1522–4.

Management of Chondral Defects Associated with Patella Instability

Mark T. Langhans, MD, PhD, Sabrina M. Strickland, MD,
Andreas H. Gomoll, MD*

KEYWORDS

- Patellofemoral • Cartilage • MACI • PJAC • Osteochondral allograft • OATS
- Chondroplasty • Patella

KEY POINTS

- Cartilage defects of the patellofemoral joint are commonly associated with patellofemoral instability events.
- Addressing the anatomic factors contributing to instability has benefits for offloading damaged cartilage.
- Defects can be addressed with cartilage repair or osteochondral techniques.

BACKGROUND

Although patellar instability overall is a relatively rare entity, it has a higher incidence in adolescents[1] and can have a lasting impairment on quality of life.[2] Importantly, in the setting of patellar dislocation, patellofemoral cartilage defects are common—patellar dislocation has been associated with chondral defects in up to 95% of patients.[3] Although the correction of any anatomic risk factors for patellar instability and risk of recurrence of instability must be addressed first, residual cartilage lesions of the patellofemoral joint are a major source of pain in these patients.[4] The inherent lack of regenerative capacity of articular cartilage combined with the high incidence of patellar instability in young populations[1] have spurred the development of several cartilage restoration procedures. The goal of these procedures is to improve the patient's pain and function by restoring the function of the patellofemoral joint cartilage as a smooth, congruent, stable, load- and shear-bearing surface.

HISTORY

Historically, osteochondral allografts (OCA) were one of the earliest attempted treatments for patellofemoral cartilage lesions. Although the first reported instance of

Hospital for Special Surgery, 535 E 70th Street, New York, NY 10021, USA
* Corresponding author.
E-mail address: gomolla@HSS.EDU

Clin Sports Med 41 (2022) 137–155
https://doi.org/10.1016/j.csm.2021.07.005
0278-5919/22/© 2021 Elsevier Inc. All rights reserved.

sportsmed.theclinics.com

OCA transplantation in the knee was in 1908, it was not until advances in the understanding of immunology and graft preservation methods in the 1970s that they became a more viable clinical option.[5] The advent of arthroscopic knee surgery in the 1970s spurred the development of several arthroscopic treatments for chondral defects including loose body removal, debridement of unstable cartilage lesions (chondroplasty), and microfracture.[6] Simultaneously, advances were being made in knee arthroplasty that made it into a viable clinical options for patients with extensive knee arthritis.[7] However, for a subset of younger patients with focal cartilage defects, treatment options remained limited.

Advances in cell culture techniques in the 1980s led to the development of the first generation of autologous chondrocyte implantation (ACI) with the first reported study in humans in 1994.[8] For limited, focal defects, arthroscopic osteochondral autograft transfer (OATs) of plugs from lesser weight-bearing areas to critical defects was first described by Matsusue and associates in 1993[9] and later popularized by Hangody and Füles.[10]

More recently, continued advances in cell culture, tissue processing, and graft preservation have led to the development of "off-the-shelf" options, including particulated juvenile allograft cartilage (PJAC; Denovo NT), micronized allograft cartilage matrix (Biocartilage), and cryopreserved, viable OCA with thin osseus layer (Prochondrix and Cartiform). The third generation of ACI incorporates a collagen matrix scaffold (MACI) and was approved for clinical use by the US Food and Drug Administration in 2016. The outcomes related to OCAs continue to improve as methods advance to preserve graft viability.[11] Similarly, continued advances in indications, design, and surgical technique have made modern onlay patellofemoral joint replacement arthroplasty an effective solution for chronic degenerative changes isolated to the patellofemoral joint.[12]

PATHOANATOMY AND BIOMECHANICS

The patellofemoral joint has a unique morphology and biomechanics that make it especially prone to instability and the development of associated chondral lesions.[13] The patella articulates with the trochlear groove, which is formed from the lateral and medial facets at the distal aspect of the femur. Although the trochlear cartilage is 3.7 mm at its thickest, the patellar cartilage at 7 mm is the thickest cartilage in the body.[14] As the largest sesamoid in the body, it is responsible for increasing the mechanical advantage of the extensor mechanism by decreasing the quadriceps force required to extend the knee.[15] This point is underscored by the finding that there is a 30% decrease in the quadriceps moment arm after patellectomy.[16] The joint reactive forces experienced at the patellofemoral joint vary greatly with different activities—up to 7.8 times body weight during a deep squat, 5.6 times body weight while running, and 3.3 times body weight while on stairs.[17,18]

Contact between the patella and trochlea is dynamic and varies depending on flexion of the knee. The patella engages in the trochlear grove at 20° to 30° of knee flexion. The lateral facet of the trochlea serves as a major restraint to lateral subluxation of the patella in conjunction with the vastus medialis, the medial patellofemoral ligament, and the medial retinaculum. In the terminal portion of extension (0°–30°), the soft tissue structures serve as the primary restraint to lateral subluxation. Beyond 30° flexion, the patella engages the trochlea, which serves as the primary restraint against lateral subluxation.[19] At low flexion angles, patellar contact points in the trochlear groove are on the central or slightly medial side and shift laterally in deeper flexion.[20] Disruption of the medial soft tissue restraints can predispose the patella to lateral dislocation, and the abnormal contact outside of the trochlear groove can result in a traumatic articular cartilage lesion, typically of the inferomedial patellar facet or the lateral femoral condyle.[21,22]

ANATOMIC RISK FACTORS FOR PATELLAR INSTABILITY AND CARTILAGE DEFECTS

Several anatomic risk factors have been identified for patellar instability events and associated patellofemoral chondral defects including trochlear dysplasia, patella alta, lateralized tibial tubercle, genu valgum, femoral anteversion, and external tibial torsion. Trochlear dysplasia has historically been classified according to the Dejour classification,[23] but more concrete measures of dysplasia are trochlear depth, lateral trochlear inclination, and facet asymmetry. Measured at 3 cm proximal to the joint line, a trochlear depth of less than 3 mm, facet asymmetry of less than 2:5 (medial:lateral),[24] or a lateral trochlear inclination angle of less than $11°$[25] were sensitive and specific measures for the diagnosis of trochlear dysplasia. Patellar height can be assessed using several different measurements including Caton–Deschamps, Insall–Salvati, and Blackburn–Peel.[26–28] A patella alta increased the height of the patella, predisposing the knee to patellar instability owing to the high flexion angle required to engage the patella in the trochlea. Lateralization of the tibial tubercle is commonly assessed by measurement of the tibial tubercle–trochlear groove distance, with a normal range of 8.9 to 11.1 mm measured on MRI.[29] A distance of greater than 20 mm is associated with increased patellar instability,[23] and a recent study suggests that patients with a tibial tubercle–trochlear groove of greater than 17 mm benefit from bony realignment to decrease this distance.[30] Other proposed measures of tibial tubercle lateralization that may perform better as predictors of patellar instability include tibial tubercle–lateral trochlear ridge distance,[31] tibial tubercle–midepicondyle distance,[32] and tibial tubercle–posterior cruciate ligament distance.[33] Coronal and rotational alignment parameters have also been shown to play an important role in patellar instability. Genu valgum,[34] femoral anteversion,[35] and external tibial torsion[36] have all been associated with patellar instability.

The importance of addressing patellar instability before or concomitantly with the chondral defect is underscored by the finding that anatomic risk factors for patellar instability are also significantly associated with the presence of patellofemoral chondral defects. A cross-sectional study of 235 patients with a history of patellofemoral instability found that the risk factors for cartilage lesions of the patellofemoral joint included a significantly higher sulcus angle, lower trochlear sulcus depth, lower angle of Fulkerson, lower patellar width, and higher Insall–Salvati ratio. Among patients with cartilage lesions, 36% had trochlear dysplasia, 27.6% patella alta, and 24.6% an abnormal tilt.[37] Similarly, a case series of 26 patients undergoing medial patellofemoral ligament reconstruction found that trochlear dysplasia was significantly associated with cartilage defects, particularly of the distal medial patella.[38] Additionally, in patients undergoing procedures for patellar instability, patellar cartilage defects were correlated with persistent pain,[39] complications, and poor outcomes.[4]

HISTORY AND PHYSICAL EXAMINATION

Patients presenting with patellar instability often, but not necessarily, endorse a complete patellar dislocation event. Important details to note are the mechanism of injury (contact or noncontact), occurrence of more than 1 subluxation or dislocation event, a history of prior surgery for patellar instability, contralateral dislocation, and the timing and resolution of the dislocations—if the patella relocated spontaneously or remain dislocated with reduction requiring sedation. The most common mechanism for first time patellar dislocation is internal rotation on a planted foot with a valgus component and the knee in early flexion.[40] Contralateral dislocation, noncontact dislocations, and recurrent dislocations are all associated with a higher risk of future dislocations.[41] In general, patients can be classified into 3 groups: first time dislocators, recurrent dislocators, and failures of prior patellar instability procedures.[42] Another important factor to note is the presence of anterior knee pain with activities that load the patellofemoral joint, namely, stair climbing, running, or deep flexion. In patients presenting with anterior knee pain, cartilage defects were found on MRI more commonly in the patella than in the trochlea.[43] The presence of mechanical symptoms such as locking or catching of the knee has been found to be correlated more closely with chondral lesions than meniscal pathology.[44]

The physical examination of a patient presenting with a history consistent with patellar instability provides critical information for guiding future imaging workup and interventions. Swelling of the knee is found in patients with acute trauma and/or intra-articular pathology, including chondral defects. The quadriceps muscles are critical to maintaining normal patella tracking, and atrophy, particularly of the vastus medialis obliquus, may be associated with patellar instability and be a target for physical therapy intervention.[45] Crepitus of the patellofemoral joint with flexion and extension of the knee is also a potential sign of chondral lesions.[46] It is important to note at what degree of flexion crepitus is noted—early flexion would indicate a lesion of the distal patella, whereas late flexion would indicate a lesion of the proximal patella. Tenderness at the lateral or medial trochlea or at the lateral or medial patellar facet is also important to note and is associated with maltracking and chondral lesions. Apprehension from the patient with laterally directed force on the patella at 0° to 30° of flexion is associated with maltracking, and translation of the patella more than 2 quadrants lateral is abnormal. The J-sign is a lateral translation of the patella as the leg is brought out to extension and the patella leaves the trochlear groove and is a sign of maltracking. Coronal deformity should be assessed as genu valgum is a risk factor for patellar instability. Other important parameters to assess include rotational parameters—excess hip internal rotation is associated with femoral anteversion, and an increased thigh–foot angle is associated with external tibial torsion.[42] Hypermobility can be assessed with the Beighton score, and is associated with patellar instability.[47]

IMAGING

Radiographic evaluation should include a standard knee series with a lateral view, bilateral weight-bearing anteroposterior views, bilateral flexed Rosenberg views, and bilateral flexed axial views (Merchant). The Merchant view (knee flexed at 30°) is the preferred view for the evaluation of subluxation, because this angle of flexion is the one at which the patella is just beginning to engage the trochlear groove. From these views, assessment of joint space narrowing, loose bodies, trochlear dysplasia, patellar tilt, patellar height, and femoral anteversion can be assessed. Full-length standing films are necessary for the measurement of leg lengths to evaluate for discrepancy as well lower limb axial alignment parameters, including coronal and sagittal alignment.[48]

MRI is the most commonly used advanced imaging modality and has excellent sensitivity for detection of capsular, ligamentous, chondral, and bony injuries associated with patellar instability. MRI also allows for measurement of several anatomic risk factors for patellar instability including measurement of tibial tubercle lateralization and trochlear dysplasia. T2-weighted sequences with fat saturation facilitate assessment of cartilage and subchondral bony edema. T1rho has shown excellent sensitivity for detecting early chondral degeneration. Important parameters to consider with knee MRI with regard to assessment of patellar instability include a sequence of thin cuts through the patellofemoral joint to closely assess cartilage, especially orthogonal imaging of the trochlea (trochlea oblique views). Other important findings on MRI include loose bodies in the gutters or pouch, associated ligament injury, the presence of effusion, and the presence of bony edema in the patella or femur consistent with patellar instability. The typical pattern of bony edema found in acute patellar dislocation is lateral femoral condyle and medial patellar facet. Bony edema in the patella in particular has been found to correlate clinically with anterior knee pain.[40] A computed tomography scan is the gold standard for the assessment of femoral anteversion and tibial torsion, but recent studies have demonstrated reliable measurement with biplanar radiography[49] and zero echo time MRI.[50]

CONSERVATIVE MANAGEMENT

The majority of chondral defects associated with patellar instability are less than 2 cm[2][51] and are managed with conservative, nonoperative treatment. First-line treatment includes physical therapy, nonsteroidal anti-inflammatory drugs, intra-articular corticosteroid injections, hyaluronic acid injections,[52] and platelet-rich plasma.[53] The use of bone marrow- and adipose-derived mesenchymal stromal cell injections have been described,[54] but are still lacking the evidence to support their regular use. Tailored physical therapy includes vastus medialis oblique training through closed chain exercises, stretching of lateral structures, patellar mobilization and taping, gluteal control, and core strengthening.[55] Physical therapy for patellar instability has been demonstrated to improve patient outcomes after 8 weeks.[56]

The optimization of modifiable factors including smoking cessation,[57] regular exercise, diet,[58] and weight loss[59] can help to preserve function and manage pain symptoms. Underscoring the importance of weight loss for unloading and preserving the patellofemoral joint, the PROOF trial (Prevention of Knee Osteoarthritis in Overweight Females) examined the effect of weight change on MRI in overweight and obese women without clinical knee ostetoarthritis. Baseline and follow-up 1.5 T MRIs were scored with the MRI Osteoarthritis Knee Score. Progression of synovitis was seen in 18% of those with weight gain versus 7% of those with stable weight. The odds ratio for patellofemoral bone marrow lesions and cartilage defects was 1.62 (95% confidence interval, 0.92–2.84) in the weight gain versus the stable weight group.[59] Patellofemoral chondral lesions are indicated for surgery with persistent pain, swelling, and mechanical symptoms after a nonoperative trial.[60]

PATELLAR INSTABILITY PROCEDURES

In patellofemoral chondral defects secondary to patellar instability, it is critical to first address the root cause of the lesion by preventing recurrence of patellar instability that could compromise any cartilage repair intervention and/or cause new injury. In patients presenting with patellar instability, 30% to 70% can expect a recurrence of instability with nonoperative management.[61,62] Surgical interventions for patellar instability should be carefully tailored to the specific anatomic risk factors with which the patient is presenting. Corrective rotational osteotomies can rarely become necessary to correct significantly abnormal femoral anteversion and external tibial torsion. Genu valgum can be corrected in adolescents with growth remaining with guided growth,[63] and in growth mature patient with an opening or closing wedge osteotomy.[34]

In the absence of any specific anatomic risk factors, medial patellofemoral ligament reconstruction has emerged as the first-line treatment for patellar instability with reliable improvements in patient-reported outcomes, return to sport, and prevention of recurrent instability.[64] Although isolated lateral release likely has little role in addressing instability, it has been shown to be effective in conjunction with other procedures and for the correction of lateral patellar tilt.[65] Recently, lateral retinacular lengthening has seen increased popularity with reported better outcomes than lateral release.

Tibial tubercle osteotomy (TTO) is a powerful tool for the correction of anatomic risk factors. Patella alta can be addressed with a distalizing TTO.[39] A lateralized tibial tubercle can be addressed with a medializing TTO. Anteriorization TTO helps to offload the patellofemoral joint.[66] The Fulkerson osteotomy is a commonly performed anteromedialization TTO that decreases lateralization of the patella[67] while simultaneously shifting contact force to the medial trochlea and decreasing contact pressure at all flexion angles.[68]

Likely because of offloading of the patellofemoral joint, studies have found that cartilage restoration techniques in the patellofemoral joint performed in conjunction with anteromedialization TTO have superior outcomes to isolated patellofemoral cartilage restoration techniques.[69-72] Another study found that anteromedialization TTO with MACI has good results at 5- to 11-year follow-up with an International Knee Documentation Committee score of 75.7 and a Lsyholm score of 79.3.[73] Additionally, a systematic review found MACI with patellofemoral osteotomy was superior to MACI alone with regard to clinical outcomes.[74] Interestingly, Pidoriano and colleagues[75] reported on 36 patients with chondral lesions of the patellofemoral joint who underwent isolated TTO with improvement in patient reported outcomes—those with distal or lateral lesions had 87% good or excellent outcomes, whereas those with medial facet lesions had 55% good or excellent outcomes, and those with proximal or diffuse patellar lesions had only 20% good or excellent outcomes.[73-75] This study suggests that the location of the lesion in the patellofemoral joint and the specific loading patterns of the joint contribute significantly to the outcome, and that alteration of the biomechanics of the patellofemoral joint can play a significant role in optimizing the environment for the patellofemoral cartilage.

CARTILAGE PROCEDURES

Operative interventions for focal chondral defects can be classified as palliative, reparative, restorative, or reconstructive.[76] Palliative procedures include the removal of loose bodies or unstable fragments or flaps of cartilage in a process known as chondroplasty. Chondroplasty is typically performed with a mechanical shaver, although there are reports of the use of radiofrequency energy devices. A systematic review of radiofrequency energy chondroplasty for the arthroscopic treatment of knee chondral lesions suggests slightly superior outcomes than with a mechanical shaver alone, potentially owing to the ability of the radiofrequency probe to anneal the exposed layers of cartilage.[77] There is a small risk of osteonecrosis of the underlying bone with radiofrequency energy, but a prospective study that used MRI at 6 months detected signs of bone osteonecrosis in only 2 of 50 patients and concluded that it could be avoided with proper surgical technique.[78]

Reparative procedures include fixation of osteochondral fragments, typically with fibrin glue,[79] sutures,[80] bioabsorbable implants,[81] or headless compression screws.[82] Fragment repair should be performed whenever possible, provided the fragment is of sufficient size and quality to allow fixation. Small defects (<2 cm^2) that are limited to the inferomedial patella or the margin of the anterior lateral femoral condyle are generally not symptomatic and can be treated with debridement alone.

Reparative techniques also include microfracture and related marrow stimulation techniques, which are typically reserved for small defects less than 2 cm^2 in size. Microfracture involves debridement of the lesion to bone, followed by the use of an awl to create bleeding perforations in the subchondral bone, allowing a fibrin clot to form that later matures to scar tissue.[83] Although patients younger than 40 years of age showed some improvement,[84] patient-reported outcome measures are worse in older patients and in the patellofemoral joint, and tend to deteriorate significantly at 18 to 36 months postoperatively.[85] Although several studies have demonstrated that microfracture has inferior outcomes compared with restorative and reconstructive techniques,[86,87] other investigators have failed to find significant differences at long-term follow-up.[88]

Several reparative adjuncts to microfracture have been developed and include platelet-rich plasma, bone marrow aspirate concentrate, and adipose-derived stem cells. Micronized cartilage extracellular matrix (Biocartilage) and PJAC represent off-the-shelf technologies that can be used with or separate from microfracture. The minced pieces of cartilage or cartilage matrix are typically mixed with a biological adjuvant such as platelet-rich plasma or bone marrow aspirate concentrate and placed into the debrided defect (**Fig. 1**). Importantly, this technique requires a dry environment, which can be difficult to facilitate arthroscopically.[89] Its use in defects up 7 cm^2 has been reported in the patellofemoral joint.[90] These technologies have been used successfully in the treatment of trochlear defects with postoperative improvement in patient-reported outcomes at 2 years and the majority of the lesions demonstrating more than 50% fill on MRI[91,92] PJAC also been used in the treatment of full-thickness patellar chondral defects, with good to excellent fill on MRI and stable

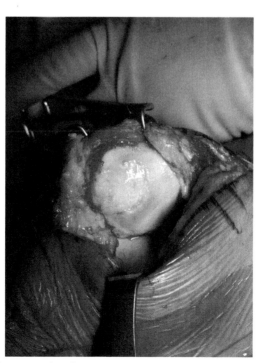

Fig. 1. Patellar defect treated with PJAC.

improvement in outcomes at 2 years.[93] It can also be used as an adjunct to fill small defects beside osteochondral autologous transfer (OAT) or OCA grafts.

ACI is a restorative technology for chondral defects. ACI is a 2-stage procedure. In the first stage, 200 to 300 mg of articular cartilage from the femoral intercondylar notch or periphery of the femoral condyles is harvested, the chondrocytes are isolated enzymatically, expanded in culture to produce a monolayer, and, historically, resuspended and sent as a cell suspension. In the current generation, termed matrix ACI (MACI), the chondrocytes are now seeded onto a collagen membrane. The surgeon receives 1 or multiple collagen membranes with cells adherent to the membrane, which is applied directly to the defect and secured with fibrin glue (**Fig. 2**) or suture anchors, or tied through bone tunnels made with K wires.[94]

MACI was approved in December 2016 by the US Food and Drug Administration for use in the treatment of symptomatic articular cartilage defects in the knee with or without bony involvement based on the results of the European SUMMIT (Superiority of MACI Implant vs Microfracture Treatment) randomized controlled trial, which showed significantly superior functional outcomes at 2 years of follow-up versus microfracture for Outerbridge III or IV lesions of the femoral condyles or trochlea greater than 3 cm^2.[86] The use of MACI for patella chondral lesions was the most commonly treated area of the knee (36.5% of cases) in the reported series of the first 1000 cases in the United States.[95]

MACI has demonstrated excellent results within the patellofemoral joint. In 1 study of patients with patellar chondral defects, 27 patients underwent MACI and 11 microfractures for a mean defect size 2.6 cm^2. At 45.1 months average follow-up, the MACI cohort reported better International Knee Documentation Committee sore, Lysholm, and Tegner scores with a lower rate of failure and lower visual analog scale.[96] In a multicenter study of 110 patients followed for an average of 7.5 years, 92% of patients reported they would undergo ACI again, and 84% remained significantly improved at final follow-up.[97] The results of these studies are reflected in clinical practice patterns, which has shown a trend in the decreased use of microfracture and an increased use of MACI for patellofemoral joint cartilage defects.[95]

The status of the subchondral bone is an important consideration in patients presenting with isolated patellofemoral cartilage defects. In 30 patients who underwent MACI, there was a negative correlation between cartilage repair tissue and subchondral bone marrow lesion volume.[98] In line with these findings, another study reported that MACI results after microfracture were inferior to those without prior microfracture.[99] Although MACI with autologous bone grafting has been reported for the

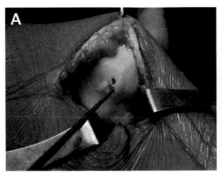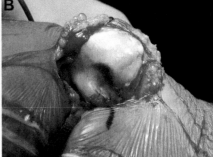

Fig. 2. Median ridge patellar cartilage defect before (*A*) and after (*B*) treatment with MACI.

femoral condyles, 7 of 21 patients had incomplete filling of the defect and 6 of those 7 had pain associated with deep bony defects and persistent underlying bone marrow edema.[100] These findings underscore the importance of the integrity of the subchondral bone to the repair of cartilage defects.

OSTEOCHONDRAL PROCEDURES

Biologic reconstructive techniques include OAT and OCA transplantation (**Fig. 3**). OAT involves the transfer of an osteochondral plug from a non–weight-bearing area, typically the non–weight-bearing portion of the trochlea in the notch into the defect. OAT is limited by donor site morbidity and availability, and it is technically challenging in the patellofemoral joint because of the unique morphology and thickness of the cartilage. One reported solution for OAT donor site morbidity is to backfill the donor site with an OCA plug.[101] Studies of patients treated with OAT for patellofemoral defects reported significant improvement in patient-reported outcomes that correlates with good fill of cartilage defects on MRI.[102] Shorter term studies have reported excellent outcomes at 1 and 2 years of follow-up.[103–105] At longer term follow-up, Hangody and colleagues[106] reported that 74% of patients had good to excellent outcomes at a mean follow-up of 9.6 years after treatment with OAT for patellofemoral lesions, but that the results were inferior to those for OAT in other areas of the knee. Solheim and colleagues[107] reported similar long-term survival at 18 years between OAT in the patellofemoral and tibiofemoral joints with 40% of patients with Lysholm scores of greater than 65 and no arthroplasty. The initial excitement for patellofemoral OAT was tempered by the report of Bentley and colleagues[108] that all 5 patellar OATs failed in their series.

Fresh OCA transplantation (**Fig. 4**) uses cadaveric plugs taken from 14- to 28-day-old donor tissue to fill chondral lesions. The initial 14 days are required for safety testing, and graft chondrocyte viability, closely associated with outcomes, has been shown to decrease significantly at 28 days.[109] OCA avoids the potential for donor site morbidity of OAT and can be helpful in matching the morphology of the patellofemoral joint with the availability of patellofemoral grafts with the tradeoff of immune

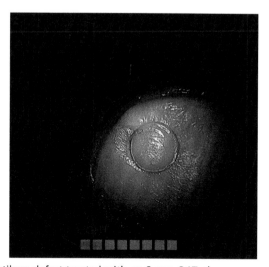

Fig. 3. Patellar cartilage defect treated with an 8-mm OAT plug.

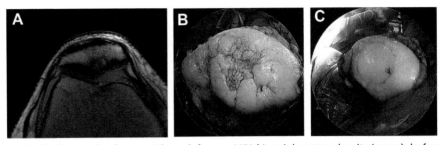

Fig. 4. Medial patellar facet cartilage defect on MRI (*A*; axial proton density image), before (*B*) and after (*C*) treatment with OCA.

mismatch. Patient-reported outcomes are similar to those for OAT and ACI in the patellofemoral joint.[110] Case series reported a 10-year survivorship of 91% in the trochlea[111] versus 78% in the patella.[112] It has been reported for bipolar lesions, including both the patella and the trochlea[113,114]

Cryopreserved, viable OCAs are chondral allografts with a wafer thin osseus backing with a regular array of perforations to facilitate penetration of the cryopreservation solution. They have a significantly longer shelf life than fresh OCAs because they can be frozen and stored.[115] Their use for the treatment of patellofemoral cartilage defects has been reported in smaller case series[116] that have shown patient-reported outcome measures comparable with other reconstructive techniques at 2 years of follow-up.[117]

Technical pearls for patellofemoral osteochondral grafts
- A compartment-matched graft is preferred to ensure appropriate thickness of the patella or trochlear articular cartilage.
- Maintain as little bone as possible on the graft, limiting the total graft thickness to 6 to 8 mm (depending on the relative thickness of cartilage in the plug).
- Be prepared to use multiple plugs in a "snowman" configuration.
- Before inserting the plugs, the recipient socket should be dilated for easier graft passage.

PATELLOFEMORAL JOINT ARTHROPLASTY

Arthroplasty represents a nonbiologic reconstructive procedure. The pathoanatomy of patellar instability leads to isolated patellofemoral chondral defects, making patients with extensive isolated patellofemoral osteoarthritis secondary to patellar instability prime candidates for unicompartmental patellofemoral arthroplasty. Although early inlay patellofemoral arthroplasty designs suffered from high failure rates, advances in design including larger onlay prostheses have corrected many of the problems that arose with regard to maltracking and catching.[76] Patellofemoral arthroplasty results in better early patient reported outcomes and range of movement versus total knee arthroplasty,[118] representing an attractive alternative to total knee arthroplasty in younger, more active patients.

POSTOPERATIVE PROTOCOL: PATELLOFEMORAL CARTILAGE AND OSTEOCHONDRAL PROCEDURES

- Stage 1 (weeks 1–6 postoperatively): Locked brace for ambulation, continuous passive motion 6 to 8 hours per day, range of motion and isometric muscle exercises. Weight bearing restricted for 6 weeks to touchdown when TTO is performed; otherwise, wight-bearing as tolerated in full extension, continuous passive motion for days 0 to 40 and advanced 5° per day (slower with larger or bipolar defects).

- Stage 2 (weeks 7–12 postoperatively): Active range of motion exercises, but avoidance of open chain knee extension and repetitive flexion knee loading.
- Stage 3 (weeks ≥12): Advance functional activities, open chain knee extension, and stair climbing are discouraged for 6 months. Restricted from inline impact activities (running) for 12 to 18 months and cutting sports for 18 months.

Early goals include decreasing pain and effusion. The graft should be protected from load and shear forces. Knee range of motion is required to decrease the incidence of arthrofibrosis, but limited to 90° to protect the surgical site. Immediate patellar mobilization in all directions is recommended to avoid scarring and adhesions. Early stage quadriceps strengthening including terminal knee extensions and straight leg raises in a knee immobilizer should be performed daily. Cryotherapy can play an important role in decreasing inflammation and associated joint effusion.[119]

OUTCOMES COMPARISON

A systematic review and meta-analysis of 14 randomized controlled trials with 775 patients found Knee injury and Osteoarthritis Outcome Score Sports and Recreation as the most responsive section of the Knee injury and Osteoarthritis Outcome Score after operative intervention for cartilage defect and noted that MACI/ACI had significantly better outcomes at 2 years versus microfracture.[120] Similarly, a systematic review of studies published from 1990 to 2018 found that patients with patellofemoral cartilage lesions treated with cartilage restoration procedures (MACI/ACI, OATS, PJAC) had significant improvements in functional outcome scores compared with preoperatively at 2 years follow-up.[121] These results correlated with moderate to complete infill of patellar cartilage lesions seen on MRI.[122]

There is a high level of evidence to support the treatment of medium sized lesions (2–4 cm^2) with OCA or OATS. These techniques are technically more demanding in the patellofemoral joint owing to its morphology. For larger lesions, the morbidity associated with OATS graft donor site precludes its use. OCAs and MACI are the preferred options for defects greater than 4 cm^2. In the setting of compromised subchondral bone, OCA may be preferred over MACI. For instances where a 2-stage MACI is not feasible or desirable, off-the-shelf options such as PJAC, micronized allograft cartilage matrix, and cryopreserved, viable OCAs may be acceptable alternatives although the evidence remains limited to date.[123]

FINAL CONSIDERATIONS

Despite their demonstrated inferiority to cartilage restoration techniques, palliative procedures dominate with regard to the management of patellofemoral chondral defects associated with patellar instability. In a review of the PearlDiver insurance database of cartilage procedures performed in the knee from 2004 to 2011 in the United States, palliative procedures dominated, and chondroplasty was by far the most common procedure (132,191), followed by microfracture (46,592). There were significantly fewer cartilage restoration procedures—OCA (605), ACI (593), and OATs (207).[124] Several practical barriers likely contribute to these findings. OCA is limited by the availability of appropriate donor tissue. MACI and OATS are limited by insurance approvals. PJAC, micronized allograft cartilage matrix, and cryopreserved, viable OCAs are gaining popularity from their ease of use and availability.

In the short term, the role for and interaction of cartilage procedures with realignment and offloading remains to be elucidated. Innovation in rehabilitation protocols will also allow improvements in patient outcomes and satisfaction. In the long term, a better understanding of the biology and immunology associated with these defects and techniques to address them will allow incremental improvements.

CLINICS CARE POINTS

- Cartilage defects of the patellofemoral joint are commonly associated with patellofemoral instability events
- Addressing anatomic factors contributing to instability also has benefits for offloading damaged cartilage
- Defects between 2 and 6 cm^2 can be addressed with cartilage repair (PJAC, MACI) or osteochondral techniques
- Patellofemoral arthroplasty for isolated patellofemoral arthritis is an alternative to total knee arthroplasty

DISCLOSURE

S. Strickland and A. Gomoll are consultants for Vericel (MACI), and Andreas Gomoll is a consultant for JRF (OCA).

REFERENCES

1. Sanders TL, Pareek A, Hewett TE, et al. Incidence of first-time lateral patellar dislocation: a 21-year population-based study. Sports Health 2018;10(2): 146–51.
2. Moström EB, Mikkelsen C, Weidenhielm L, et al. Long-term follow-up of nonoperatively and operatively treated acute primary patellar dislocation in skeletally immature patients. Sci World J 2014;2014. https://doi.org/10.1155/2014/473281.
3. Kita K, Tanaka Y, Toritsuka Y, et al. Patellofemoral chondral status after medial patellofemoral ligament reconstruction using second-look arthroscopy in patients with recurrent patellar dislocation. J Orthop Sci 2014;19(6):925–32.
4. Dalal S, Setia P, Debnath A, et al. Recurrent patellar dislocations with patellar cartilage defects: a pain in the knee? Knee 2021;29:55–62.
5. Nikolaou VS, Giannoudis PV. History of osteochondral allograft transplantation. Injury 2017;48(7):1283–6.
6. Hunt SA, Jazrawi LM, Sherman OH. Arthroscopic management of osteoarthritis of the knee. J Am Acad Orthop Surg 2002;10(5):356–63.
7. Papas PV, Cushner FD, Scuderi GR. The history of total knee arthroplasty. Tech Orthop 2018;33(1):2–6.
8. Brittberg M, Lindahl A, Nilsson A, et al. N Engl J Med 1994;331(14):889–95.
9. Matsusue Y, Yamamuro T, Hama H. Arthroscopic multiple osteochondral transplantation to the chondral defect in the knee associated with anterior cruciate ligament disruption. Arthroscopy 1993;9(3):318–21.
10. Hangody L, Füles P. Autologous osteochondral mosaicplasty for the treatment of full-thickness defects of weight-bearing joints: ten years of experimental and clinical experience. J Bone Joint Surg Am 2003;85(SUPPL. 1):25–32.
11. Hevesi M, Denbeigh JM, Paggi CA, et al. Fresh osteochondral allograft transplantation in the knee: a viability and histologic analysis for optimizing graft viability and expanding existing standard processed graft resources using a

living donor cartilage program. Cartilage 2019. https://doi.org/10.1177/1947603519880330.

12. Pisanu G, Rosso F, Bertolo C, et al. Patellofemoral arthroplasty: current concepts and review of the literature. Joints 2017;5(4):237–45.

13. Baumann CA, Hinckel BB, Tanaka MJ. Update on patellofemoral anatomy and biomechanics. Oper Tech Sports Med 2019;27(4):150683.

14. Cohen ZA, Mow VC, Henry JH, et al. Templates of the cartilage layers of the patellofemoral joint and their use in the assessment of osteoarthritic cartilage damage. Osteoarthr Cartil 2003;11(8):569–79.

15. Grelsamer RP, Weinstein CH. Applied biomechanics of the patella. Clin Orthop Relat Res 2001;389(389):9–14.

16. Kaufer H. Mechanical function of the patella. J Bone Joint Surg Am 1971;53(8):1551–60.

17. Loudon JK. Biomechanics and pathomechanics of the patellofemoral joint. Int J Sports Phys Ther 2016;11(6):820–30.

18. Flynn TW, Soutas-Little RW. Patellofemoral joint compressive forces in forward and backward running. J Orthop Sports Phys Ther 1995;21(5):277–82.

19. Kane PW, Tucker BS, Frederick R, et al. Cartilage restoration of the patellofemoral joint. JBJS Rev 2017;5(10). https://doi.org/10.2106/JBJS.RVW.17.00020.

20. Suzuki T, Hosseini A, Li JS, et al. In vivo patellar tracking and patellofemoral cartilage contacts during dynamic stair ascending. J Biomech 2012;45(14):2432–7.

21. Farr J, Covell DJ, Lattermann C. Cartilage lesions in patellofemoral dislocations: incidents/locations/when to treat. Sports Med Arthrosc 2012;20(3):181–6.

22. Nomura E, Inoue M, Kurimura M. Chondral and osteochondral injuries associated with acute patellar dislocation. Arthroscopy 2003;19(7):717–21.

23. Dejour H, Walch G, Nove-Josserand L, et al. Factors of patellar instability: an anatomic radiographic study. *Knee Surgery.* Sport Traumatol Arthrosc 1994;2(1):19–26.

24. Pfirrmann CWA, Zanetti M, Romero J, et al. Femoral trochlear dysplasia: MR findings. Radiology 2000;216(3):858–64.

25. Carrillon Y, Abidi H, Dejour D, et al. Patellar instability: assessment on MR images by measuring the lateral trochlear inclination - Initial experience. Radiology 2000;216(2):582–5.

26. Yanke AB, Wuerz T, Saltzman BM, et al. Management of patellofemoral chondral injuries. Clin Sports Med 2014;33(3):477–500.

27. Aglietti P, Insall JN, Cerulli G. Patellar pain and incongruence. I: measurements of incongruence. Clin Orthop Relat Res 1983;176:217–24.

28. Murray TF, Dupont J-Y, Fulkerson JP. Axial and lateral radiographs in evaluating patellofemoral malalignment. Am J Sports Med 1999;27(5):580–4.

29. Pandit S, Frampton C, Stoddart J, et al. Magnetic resonance imaging assessment of tibial tuberosity-trochlear groove distance: normal values for males and females. Int Orthop 2011;35(12):1799–803.

30. Franciozi CE, Ambra LF, Albertoni LJB, et al. Anteromedial tibial tubercle osteotomy improves results of medial patellofemoral ligament reconstruction for recurrent patellar instability in patients with tibial tuberosity–trochlear groove distance of 17 to 20 mm. Arthroscopy 2019;35(2):566–74.

31. Weltsch D, Chan CT, Mistovich RJ, et al. Predicting risk of recurrent patellofemoral instability with measurements of extensor mechanism containment. Am J Sports Med 2021;49(3):706–12.

32. Iseki T, Nakayama H, Daimon T, et al. Tibial tubercle–midepicondyle distance can be a better index to predict the outcome of medial patellofemoral ligament reconstruction than tibial tubercle-trochlear groove distance. Arthrosc Sport Med Rehabil 2020;2(6):e697–704.

33. Brady JM, Rosencrans AS, Shubin Stein BE. Use of TT-PCL versus TT-TG. Curr Rev Musculoskelet Med 2018;11(2):261–5.

34. Kwon JH, Kim JI, Seo DH, et al. Patellar dislocation with genu valgum treated by DFO. Orthopedics 2013;36(6):840–3.

35. Zhang ZJ, Zhang H, Song GY, et al. Increased femoral anteversion is associated with inferior clinical outcomes after MPFL reconstruction and combined tibial tubercle osteotomy for the treatment of recurrent patellar instability. Knee Surgery, Sport Traumatol Arthrosc 2020;28(7):2261–9.

36. Cameron JC, Saha S. External tibial torsion. Clin Orthop Relat Res 1996;328: 177–84.

37. Ambra LF, Hinckel BB, Arendt EA, et al. Anatomic risk factors for focal cartilage lesions in the patella and trochlea: a case-control study. Am J Sports Med 2019; 47(10):2444–53.

38. Holliday CL, Hiemstra LA, Kerslake S, et al. Relationship between anatomical risk factors, articular cartilage lesions, and patient outcomes following medial patellofemoral ligament reconstruction. Cartilage 2019. https://doi.org/10. 1177/1947603519894728. 1947603519894728.

39. Leite CBG, Santos TP, Giglio PN, et al. Tibial tubercle osteotomy with distalization is a safe and effective procedure for patients with patella alta and patellar instability. Orthop J Sport Med 2021;9(1). 2325967120975101.

40. Diederichs G, Issever AS, Scheffler S. MR imaging of patellar instability: injury patterns and assessment of risk factors. Radiographics 2010;30(4):961–81.

41. Fithian DC, Paxton EW, Stone M, et al. Epidemiology and natural history of acute patellar dislocation. Am J Sports Med 2004;32(5):1114–21.

42. Khan N, Stewart R, Fithian DC. Evaluation of the patient with patellar instability. Ann Jt 2018;3:56.

43. Boegård TL, Rudling O, Petersson IF, et al. Distribution of MR-detected cartilage defects of the patellofemoral joint in chronic knee pain. Osteoarthr Cartil 2003; 11(7):494–8.

44. Farina EM, Lowenstein NA, Chang Y, et al. Meniscal and mechanical symptoms are associated with cartilage damage, not meniscal pathology. J Bone Joint Surg Am 2021;103(5):381–8.

45. Smith TO, Chester R, Cross J, et al. Rehabilitation following first-time patellar dislocation: A randomised controlled trial of purported vastus medialis obliquus muscle versus general quadriceps strengthening exercises. Knee 2015;22(4): 313–20.

46. Schiphof D, Van Middelkoop M, De Klerk BM, et al. Crepitus is a first indication of patellofemoral osteoarthritis (and not of tibiofemoral osteoarthritis). Osteoarthr Cartil 2014;22(5):631–8.

47. Nomura E, Inoue M, Kobayashi S. Generalized joint laxity and contralateral patellar hypermobility in unilateral recurrent patellar dislocators. Arthroscopy 2006;22(8):861–5.

48. Sherman SL, Raines BT, Burch MB, et al. Patellofemoral imaging and analysis. Oper Tech Sports Med 2019;27(4):150684.

49. Rosskopf AB, Ramseier LE, Sutter R, et al. Femoral and tibial torsion measurement in children and adolescents: comparison of 3D models based on low-dose

biplanar radiography and low-dose CT. Am J Roentgenol 2014;202(3). https://doi.org/10.2214/AJR.13.11103.

50. Breighner RE, Bogner EA, Lee SC, et al. Evaluation of osseous morphology of the hip using zero echo time magnetic resonance imaging. Am J Sports Med 2019;47(14):3460–8.

51. Luhmann SJ, Schoenecker PL, Dobbs MB, et al. Arthroscopic findings at the time of patellar realignment surgery in adolescents. J Pediatr Orthop 2007; 27(5):493–8.

52. Strauss EJ, Galos DK. The evaluation and management of cartilage lesions affecting the patellofemoral joint. Curr Rev Musculoskelet Med 2013;6(2):141–9.

53. Chen P, Huang L, Ma Y, et al. Intra-articular platelet-rich plasma injection for knee osteoarthritis: a summary of meta-analyses. J Orthop Surg Res 2019; 14(1):385.

54. Lubis AMT, Panjaitan T, Hoo C. Autologous mesenchymal stem cell application for cartilage defect in recurrent patellar dislocation: a case report. Int J Surg Case Rep 2019;55:183–6.

55. McConnell J. The physical therapist's approach to patellofemoral disorders. Clin Sports Med 2002;21(3):363–87.

56. Chiu JKW, Wong Y, Yung PSH, et al. The effects of quadriceps strengthening on pain, function, and patellofemoral joint contact area in persons with patellofemoral pain. Am J Phys Med Rehabil 2012;91(2):98–106.

57. Amin S, Niu J, Guermazi A, et al. Cigarette smoking and the risk for cartilage loss and knee pain in men with knee osteoarthritis. Ann Rheum Dis 2007; 66(1):18–22.

58. Dean E, Gormsen Hansen R. Prescribing optimal nutrition and physical activity as "first-line" interventions for best practice management of chronic low-grade inflammation associated with osteoarthritis: evidence synthesis. Arthritis 2012; 2012:1–28.

59. Landsmeer MLA, de Vos BC, van der Plas P, et al. Effect of weight change on progression of knee OA structural features assessed by MRI in overweight and obese women. Osteoarthr Cartil 2018;26(12):1666–74.

60. Gomoll AH, Probst C, Farr J, et al. Use of a type I/III bilayer collagen membrane decreases reoperation rates for symptomatic hypertrophy after autologous chondrocyte implantation. Am J Sports Med 2009;37(Suppl 1):20S–3S.

61. Palmu S, Kallio PE, Donell ST, et al. Acute patellar dislocation in children and adolescents: a randomized clinical trial. J Bone Joint Surg Am 2008;90(3):463–70.

62. Askenberger M, Bengtsson Moström E, Ekström W, et al. Operative repair of medial patellofemoral ligament injury versus knee brace in children with an acute first-time traumatic patellar dislocation: a randomized controlled trial. Am J Sports Med 2018;46(10):2328–40.

63. Parikh SN, Redman C, Gopinathan NR. Simultaneous treatment for patellar instability and genu valgum in skeletally immature patients: a preliminary study. J Pediatr Orthop B 2019;28(2):132–8.

64. Erickson BJ, Nguyen J, Gasik K, et al. Isolated medial patellofemoral ligament reconstruction for patellar instability regardless of tibial tubercle-trochlear groove distance and patellar height: outcomes at 1 and 2 years. Am J Sports Med 2019;47(6):1331–7.

65. da Fonseca LPRM, Kawatake EH, de Pochini AC. Lateral patellar retinacular release: changes over the last ten years. Rev Bras Ortop (English Ed 2017; 52(4):442–9.

66. Rue JPH, Colton A, Zare SM, et al. Trochlear contact pressures after straight anteriorization of the tibial tuberosity. Am J Sports Med 2008;36(10):1953–9.
67. Fulkerson JP. Anteromedialization of the tibial tuberosity for patellofemoral malalignment. Clin Orthop Relat Res 1983;177:176–81.
68. Beck PR, Thomas AL, Farr J, et al. Trochlear contact pressures after anteromedialization of the tibial tubercle. Am J Sports Med 2005;33(11):1710–5.
69. Cotter EJ, Waterman BR, Kelly MP, et al. Multiple osteochondral allograft transplantation with concomitant tibial tubercle osteotomy for multifocal chondral disease of the knee. Arthrosc Tech 2017;6(4):e1393–8.
70. Farr J. Autologous chondrocyte implantation improves patellofemoral cartilage treatment outcomes. Clin Orthop Relat Res 2007;463:187–94.
71. Pritsch T, Haim A, Arbel R, et al. Tailored tibial tubercle transfer for patellofemoral malalignment: analysis of clinical outcomes. Knee Surg Sport Traumatol Arthrosc 2007;15(8):994–1002.
72. Palmer SH, Servant CT, Maguire J, et al. Surgical reconstruction of severe patellofemoral maltracking. Clin Orthop Relat Res 2004;419:144–8.
73. Gillogly SD, Arnold RM. Autologous chondrocyte implantation and anteromedialization for isolated patellar articular cartilage lesions: 5- to 11-year follow-up. Am J Sports Med 2014;42(4):912–20.
74. Trinh TQ, Harris JD, Siston RA, et al. Improved outcomes with combined autologous chondrocyte implantation and patellofemoral osteotomy versus isolated autologous chondrocyte implantation. Arthroscopy 2013;29(3):566–74.
75. Pidoriano AJ, Weinstein RN, Buuck DA, et al. Correlation of patellar articular lesions with results from anteromedial tibial tubercle transfer. Am J Sports Med 1997;25(4):533–7.
76. Otlans P, Lattermann C, Sherman SL, et al. Cartilage disease of the patellofemoral joint: realignment, restoration, replacement. Instr Course Lect 2021;70: 289–308.
77. Rocco P, Lorenzo DB, Guglielmo T, et al. Radiofrequency energy in the arthroscopic treatment of knee chondral lesions: a systematic review. Br Med Bull 2016;117(1):149–56.
78. Cetik O, Cift H, Comert B, et al. Risk of osteonecrosis of the femoral condyle after arthroscopic chondroplasty using radiofrequency: a prospective clinical series. Knee Surgery. Sport Traumatol Arthrosc 2009;17(1):24–9.
79. Visuri T, Kuusela T. Fixation of large osteochondral fractures of the patella with fibrin adhesive system: a report of two operative cases. Am J Sports Med 1989;17(6):842–5.
80. Pritsch M, Velkes S, Levy O, et al. Suture fixation of osteochondral fractures of the patella. J Bone Joint Surg Br 1995;77(1):154–5.
81. Schlechter JA, Nguyen SV, Fletcher KL. Utility of bioabsorbable fixation of osteochondral lesions in the adolescent knee: outcomes analysis with minimum 2-year follow-up. Orthop J Sport Med 2019;7(10):12–4.
82. Aydoğmuş S, Duymuş TM, Keçeci T. An unexpected complication after headless compression screw fixation of an osteochondral fracture of patella. Case Rep Orthop 2016;2016:1–4.
83. Steadman JR, Briggs KK, Rodrigo JJ, et al. Outcomes of microfracture for traumatic chondral defects of the knee: average 11-year follow-up. Arthroscopy 2003;19(5):477–84.
84. Smoak JB, Kluczynski MA, Bisson LJ, et al. Systematic review of patient outcomes and associated predictors after microfracture in the patellofemoral joint. J Am Acad Orthop Surg Glob Res Rev 2019;3(11). e10.5435.

85. Kreuz PC, Erggelet C, Steinwachs MR, et al. Is microfracture of chondral defects in the knee associated with different results in patients aged 40 years or younger? Arthroscopy 2006;22(11):1180–6.

86. Saris D, Price A, Widuchowski W, et al. Matrix-applied characterized autologous cultured chondrocytes versus microfracture: two-year follow-up of a prospective randomized trial. Am J Sports Med 2014;42(6):1384–94.

87. Solheim E, Hegna J, Strand T, et al. Randomized study of long-term (15-17 years) outcome after microfracture versus mosaicplasty in knee articular cartilage defects. Am J Sports Med 2018;46(4):826–31.

88. Knutsen G, Drogset JO, Engebretsen L, et al. A randomized multicenter trial comparing autologous chondrocyte implantation with microfracture: long-term follow-up at 14 to 15 years. J Bone Joint Surg Am 2016;98(16):1332–9.

89. Mirzayan R, Cooper JD, Chahla J. Carbon dioxide insufflation of the knee in the treatment of full-thickness chondral defects with micronized human articular cartilage. Arthrosc Tech 2018;7(10):e969–73.

90. Buckwalter JA, Bowman GN, Albright JP, et al. Clinical outcomes of patellar chondral lesions treated with juvenile particulated cartilage allografts. Iowa Orthop J 2014;34:44–9.

91. Farr J, Yao JQ. Chondral defect repair with particulated juvenile cartilage allograft. Cartilage 2011;2(4):346–53.

92. Brusalis CM, Greditzer HG, Fabricant PD, et al. BioCartilage augmentation of marrow stimulation procedures for cartilage defects of the knee: two-year clinical outcomes. Knee 2020;27(5):1418–25.

93. Grawe B, Burge A, Nguyen J, et al. Cartilage regeneration in full-thickness patellar chondral defects treated with particulated juvenile articular allograft cartilage: an MRI analysis. Cartilage 2017;8(4):374–83.

94. Ackermann J, Cole BJ, Gomoll AH. Cartilage restoration in the patellofemoral joint: techniques and outcomes. Oper Tech Sports Med 2019;27(4):150692.

95. Carey JL, Remmers AE, Flanigan DC. Use of MACI (autologous cultured chondrocytes on porcine collagen membrane) in the United States: preliminary experience. Orthop J Sport Med 2020;8(8):1–7.

96. Migliorini F, Eschweiler J, Maffulli N, et al. Management of patellar chondral defects with autologous matrix induced chondrogenesis (AMIC) compared to microfractures: a four years follow-up clinical trial. Life 2021;11(2):1–11.

97. Gomoll AH, Gillogly SD, Cole BJ, et al. Autologous chondrocyte implantation in the patella: a multicenter experience. Am J Sports Med 2014;42(5):1074–81.

98. Lyu J, Zhang Y, Zhu W, et al. Correlation between the subchondral bone marrow lesions and cartilage repair tissue after matrix-associated autologous chondrocyte implantation in the knee: a cross-sectional study. Acta Radiol 2020.

99. Minas T, Gomoll AH, Rosenberger R, et al. Increased failure rate of autologous chondrocyte implantation after previous treatment with marrow stimulation techniques. Am J Sports Med 2009;37(5):902–8.

100. Jung M, Karampinos DC, Holwein C, et al. Quantitative 3-T magnetic resonance imaging after matrix-associated autologous chondrocyte implantation with autologous bone grafting of the knee: the importance of subchondral bone parameters. Am J Sports Med 2021;49(2):476–86.

101. Vellios EE, Jones KJ, Williams RJ. Osteochondral autograft transfer for focal cartilage lesions of the knee with donor-site back-fill using precut osteochondral allograft plugs and micronized extracellular cartilage augmentation. Arthrosc Tech 2021;10(1):e181–92.

102. Nho SJ, Li F, Green DM, et al. Magnetic resonance imaging and clinical evaluation of patellar resurfacing with press-fit osteochondral autograft plugs. Am J Sports Med 2008;36(6):1101–9.
103. Astur DC, Arliani GG, Binz M, et al. Autologous osteochondral transplantation for treating patellar chondral injuries: evaluation, treatment, and outcomes of a two-year follow-up study. J Bone Joint Surg Am 2014;96(10):816–23.
104. Figueroa D, Calvo Rodriguez R, Donoso R, et al. High-grade patellar chondral defects: promising results from management with osteochondral autografts. Orthop J Sport Med 2020;8(7):1–7.
105. Emre TY, Atbasi Z, Demircioglu DT, et al. Autologous osteochondral transplantation (mosaicplasty) in articular cartilage defects of the patellofemoral joint: retrospective analysis of 33 cases. Musculoskelet Surg 2017;101(2):133–8.
106. Hangody LRL, Dobos J, Balo E, et al. Clinical experiences with autologous osteochondral mosaicplasty in an athletic population. Am J Sports Med 2010; 38(6):1125–33.
107. Solheim E, Hegna J, Inderhaug E. Clinical outcome after mosaicplasty of knee articular cartilage defects of patellofemoral joint versus tibiofemoral joint. J Orthop 2020;18:36–40.
108. Bentley G, Biant LC, Carrington RWJ, et al. A prospective, randomised comparison of autologous chondrocyte implantation versus mosaicplasty for osteochondral defects in the knee. J Bone Joint Surg Br 2003;85-B(2):223–30.
109. Cook JL, Stannard JP, Stoker AM, et al. Importance of donor chondrocyte viability for osteochondral allografts. Am J Sports Med 2016;44(5):1260–8.
110. Chahla J, Sweet MC, Okoroha KR, et al. Osteochondral allograft transplantation in the patellofemoral joint: a systematic review. Am J Sports Med 2018;47(12): 3009–18.
111. Cameron JI, Pulido PA, McCauley JC, et al. Osteochondral allograft transplantation of the femoral trochlea. Am J Sports Med 2016;44(3):633–8.
112. Gracitelli GC, Meric G, Pulido PA, et al. Fresh osteochondral allograft transplantation for isolated patellar cartilage injury. Am J Sports Med 2015;43(4):879–84.
113. Meric G, Gracitelli GC, Görtz S, et al. Fresh osteochondral allograft transplantation for bipolar reciprocal osteochondral lesions of the knee. Am J Sports Med 2015;43(3):709–14.
114. Jalali O, Vredenburgh Z, Prodromo J, et al. Bipolar fresh osteochondral allograft transplantation and joint reconstruction for patellar and trochlear cartilage defects. Arthrosc Tech 2019;8(12):e1533–41.
115. Geraghty S, Kuang JQ, Yoo D, et al. A novel, cryopreserved, viable osteochondral allograft designed to augment marrow stimulation for articular cartilage repair. J Orthop Surg Res 2015;10(1):1–13.
116. Woodmass JM, Melugin HP, Wu IT, et al. Viable osteochondral allograft for the treatment of a full-thickness cartilage defect of the patella. Arthrosc Tech 2017;6(5):e1661–5.
117. Bennett CH, Nadarajah V, Moore MC, et al. Cartiform implantation for focal cartilage defects in the knee: a 2-year clinical and magnetic resonance imaging follow-up study. J Orthop 2021;24:135–44.
118. Odgaard A, Madsen F, Kristensen PW, et al. The Mark Coventry Award: patellofemoral arthroplasty results in better range of movement and early patient-reported outcomes than TKA. Clin Orthop Relat Res 2018;476(1):87–100.
119. Bleakley C, McDonough S, MacAuley D. The use of ice in the treatment of acute soft-tissue injury: a systematic review of randomized controlled trials. Am J Sports Med 2004;32(1):251–61.

120. Abraamyan T, Johnson AJ, Wiedrick J, et al. Marrow stimulation has relatively inferior patient-reported outcomes in cartilage restoration surgery of the knee a systematic review and meta-analysis of randomized controlled trials. Am J Sports Med 2021;1–9. https://doi.org/10.1177/03635465211003595.
121. Andrade R, Nunes J, Hinckel BB, et al. Cartilage restoration of patellofemoral lesions: a systematic review. Cartilage 2019. https://doi.org/10.1177/1947603519893076.
122. Su CA, Trivedi NN, Le H, et al. Clinical and radiographic outcomes after treatment of patellar chondral defects: a systemic review. Sports Health 2021; XX(X):1–12.
123. Hinckel BB, Thomas D, Vellios EE, et al. Algorithm for treatment of focal cartilage defects of the knee: classic and new procedures. Cartilage 2021. https://doi.org/10.1177/1947603521993219.
124. McCormick F, Harris JD, Abrams GD, et al. Trends in the surgical treatment of articular cartilage lesions in the United States: an analysis of a large private-payer database over a period of 8 years. Arthroscopy 2014;30(2):222–6.

Medial Patellofemoral Ligament Repair or Medial Advancement: Is There a Role?

Iain R. Murray, MD, PhD, Christopher M. LaPrade, MD,
William Michael Pullen, MD, Seth L. Sherman, MD*

KEYWORDS

• MPFL repair • Patella dislocation • Patella instability • MPFL reconstruction

KEY POINTS

- Patella instability encompasses a broad spectrum of pathology with variable chronicity, underlying native anatomy, and concomitant injuries.
- Many surgical procedures have been proposed to address functional deficiency of the medial soft tissue restraints to patella dislocation.
- Medial patellofemoral ligament (MPFL) repair has many theoretic advantages over MPFL reconstruction and nonanatomical approaches. However, its widespread use is not supported by the more recent clinical literature.
- Current understanding on the role of MPFL repair remains limited by a lack of high-level evidence as well as numerous complex variables influencing decision making.
- High-quality, multicenter randomized controlled trials, particularly comparing MPFL repair with MPFL reconstruction while controlling for underlying risk factors are needed.

INTRODUCTION

Patellar instability is one of the most prevalent knee disorders, with dislocations occurring in 5 to 43 cases per 10,000 annually.[1,2] Traumatic patellar dislocation can result in significant morbidity and is associated with patellofemoral chondral injuries and fractures, medial soft tissue disruption, pain, and reduced function, and can lead to patellofemoral osteoarthritis. Chronic and recurrent instability can lead to deformation and incompetence of the medial soft tissue stabilizers. Despite recent gains in understanding the pathoanatomy of this disorder, the management of patients with this condition is complex and remains enigmatic.

Patellofemoral instability represents a spectrum of injuries with numerous complex patient, joint and surgeon variables influencing treatment decision making.[3–7]

Department of Orthopaedic Surgery, Stanford University, Stanford, CA, USA
* Corresponding author. Department of Orthopaedic Surgery, Stanford University, Palo Alto, CA.
E-mail address: dr.seth.sherman@gmail.com

Clin Sports Med 41 (2022) 157–169
https://doi.org/10.1016/j.csm.2021.07.006
0278-5919/22/© 2021 Elsevier Inc. All rights reserved.

Although most prevalent in skeletally immature patients, patellar instability can manifest in adults with a range of predisposing anatomic variables including limb malalignment, patellar and trochlear dysplasia, tuberosity malalignment, patella alta, and soft tissue deformation.[3–7] The medial patellofemoral ligament (MPFL) acts as the primary restraint to lateral translation of the patella.[8] Injury to the MPFL is the quintessential lesion of acute patellar dislocations, occurring in almost 100% of cases.[9–11] In this setting, MPFL disruption has been shown to occur in multiple locations with implications for surgical decision-making. Based on MRI data, Zhang and colleagues[12] reported that isolated femoral avulsion occurred in 32%, isolated patellar avulsion occurred in 39%, and ligament stretch occurred in 4%. Of note, the MPFL was disrupted in multiple locations in 25% of cases. Askenberger and colleagues[9] reported a preponderance of patellar avulsions, but also reported multifocal injuries in 35% of injuries. In contrast, Sallay and colleagues[11] found that femoral insertion site of the MPFL was injured in 87% of patients after acute patellar dislocation in their series.

Although patellar instability has traditionally been managed nonoperatively, operative interventions have gained in popularity. Multiple surgical strategies have been proposed including soft tissue and/or bony procedures. MPFL repair and reconstruction are commonly performed to address medial soft tissue deficiency in both acute[5] and recurrent patellar dislocations.[13] However, the role of MPFL repair remains controversial and there is growing literature to support the use of MPFL reconstruction.[14,15] In this review, we describe the historical evolution of medial soft tissue surgical strategies including those that seek to gain stability by altering native medial-sided knee anatomy and those that seek to restore the normal structure of the MPFL. We discuss the potential limited role for MPFL repair following acute patellar dislocation in patients with an operative osteochondral injury, normal underlying bony anatomy, and good soft tissue quality for repair. We also consider another role for MPFL repair as a soft tissue balancing procedure in patients undergoing concomitant bony procedure (ie, tibial tubercle osteotomy) for chronic patellofemoral instability.

NOMENCLATURE

Nomenclature to describe aspects of patella instability and the procedures used to treat this condition are heterogeneous and can result in ambiguity when appraising the clinical literature. For clarity, we have defined some terminology relating to pathology and management. Patella instability can broadly be divided into patients with an acute first-time subluxation/dislocation and those suffering from recurrent instability events. In acute-on chronic subluxation/dislocation events, acute tearing of already abnormal medial-sided structures occurs with or without concomitant osteochondral lesions.

Heterogeneous terms have been used to describe procedures to address patella instability. Medial-based soft tissue procedures in both acute and chronic instability settings can be divided into anatomic and nonanatomic procedures (**Table 1**). Anatomic procedures seek to restore or replace normal anatomy, whereas nonanatomic procedures seek to establish stability by modifying medial soft tissue anatomy to prevent dislocation.

First, MPFL repair is an anatomic procedure that in the acute setting seeks to restore MPFL continuity by reapproximating torn ends of the ligament in its mid substance or by reducing and securing the MPFL at its patella or femoral insertions. In the chronic setting, MPFL repair may also refer to the retensioning of a patulous MPFL that has become deformed through recurrent instability events. For completion, MPFL reconstruction is also considered an anatomic procedure, as it seeks to recreate native MPFL anatomy through the addition of a tendon graft.

Table 1
Medial-based soft tissue procedures to address patellar instability

Acute or First Time Traumatic Dislocation		Recurrent/Chronic	
Anatomic	Nonanatomic	Anatomic	Nonanatomic
MPFL Repair	None	MPFL Repair	Vastus Medialis Plasty
MPFL Reconstruction		MPFL Reconstruction	Medial Retinaculum Plication/Reefing
			Semitendinosus Tenodesis

There is also a lack of uniformity in terminology regarding each procedure. This includes medial retinaculum plication, also commonly referred to as imbrication or reefing, in which the medial soft tissues are tightened without requiring donor grafts.[16–23] Vastus medialis plasty, also referred to as medial patellar retinaculum plasty, involves distalizing and lateralizing the vastus medialis to the medial patella.[19,20,22] Lastly, for a semitendinosus tenodesis, first described by Galeazzi[24] in 1922, the proximal aspect of the semitendinosus tendon is passed obliquely across the patella.[25,26] Each of these procedures will be further described in the following section.

HISTORIC PERSPECTIVE: NONANATOMIC MEDIAL-BASED SOFT TISSUE PROCEDURES

Nonanatomic medial-based soft tissue procedures have typically been used in the setting of recurrent instability.[17] In contrast to anatomic procedures, such as MPFL repair or reconstruction, there is not an attempt to directly restore native anatomy but instead to balance the medial and lateral soft tissues.[23]

Medial Retinaculum Plication/Reefing

Medial retinaculum (or capsular) plication has been referred to as many different terms in the literature including reefing or imbrication. In contrast to MPFL repair, where the MPFL is specifically targeted and repaired, these nonanatomic procedures generally imbricate all layers indiscriminately. Although initially described as an open procedure, arthroscopic or arthroscopic-assisted techniques subsequently gained popularity.[27] The rationale was to achieve stability without requiring donor graft harvesting and donor site morbidity.[16] Proponents of this technique recommend that it be performed in patients without trochlear dysplasia, patella alta, tibial tubercle to trochlear groove distance (TT-TG) >20 mm, congenital dislocation, or hypermobility syndrome that have failed nonoperative measures.[16,18,21]

Many reports in the literature involve an arthroscopic or arthroscopic-assisted technique with a concomitant arthroscopic lateral release[18,19,27,28] although other authors have described arthroscopic techniques without lateral release.[16,19,21] There is considerable variation in the techniques described to achieve the plication. In each case, the medial retinaculum is divided and then advanced to the medial border of the patella.[16,18] Described strategies include using a suture anchor[29] in the medial patella versus mattress sutures in a "pants over vest" type of configuration.[18,19,21,27]

Vastus Medialis Plasty

Vastus medialis plasty, also referred to as medial patellar retinaculum plasty, was proposed as an alternative to the medial retinaculum plication given reports of continued instability in early studies.[20,28,29] Cited advantages include the physeal sparing nature of this technique and the increased thickness and decreased length of the medial retinaculum, thereby increasing tension to prevent lateral subluxation of the patella.[20,28,29] As with medial retinaculum plication, proponents have typically recommended this procedure in patients without constitutional laxity or skeletal risk factors for recurrence.[20,28,29]

Vastus medialis plasty involves a longitudinal incision along the medial patella in addition to a transverse incision and dissection to divide the vastus medialis and medial retinaculum. The medial retinaculum, which includes the MPFL, is then pulled proximally and laterally and sutured to the patella. Next, the vastus medialis is pulled distally and laterally and attached to the middle aspect of the patella. Following inspection of patellar tracking, the tensioning of the 2 separate limbs is adjusted and the overlapping tissues of the medial retinaculum and vastus medialis are then sutured together.[20,28,29]

Semitendinosus Tenodesis

The semitendinosus tenodesis technique was first described by Galeazzi in 1922, as a way to stabilize the patella without requiring bony stabilization. There has been a paucity of recent studies regarding this technique; however, Grannatt and colleagues[26] investigated the procedure with a modification from the original Galeazzi technique. These authors describe the indications for this procedure as recurrent patellar subluxation or dislocation in skeletally immature patients after a failure of nonoperative management.[26]

In contrast to the original description by Galeazzi, Grannatt and colleagues[26] described a modification of the semitendinosus tenodesis technique. Following diagnostic arthroscopy, a lateral release is performed in the standard fashion. A longitudinal incision is then made over the pes anserine bursa with identification of the semitendinosus tendon. While leaving the distal aspect attached, the rest of the tendon is detached from the muscle belly using a tendon stripper. A small incision is then made at the inferomedial aspect of the patella and an oblique tunnel is drilled across the patella. A superolateral incision in reference to the patella is then created to confirm the position of the tunnel. Lastly, the free end of the semitendinosus tendon graft is then passed inferomedial to superolateral through the patella and then passed back anteriorly over the patella. If any persistent patellar instability is noted on inspection, a medial retinaculum plication may then be performed.[26]

Outcomes for Medial-Based Soft Tissue Procedures

Many case series have investigated the outcomes of medial-based soft tissue procedures. These case series reported promising outcomes after medial retinaculum plication in terms of clinical outcomes measures and radiographic measures (including congruence angle, lateral patellofemoral angle, and lateral patellar displacement),[16,21,27,30] although these studies did have contrasting results in regards to recurrence of dislocations.[16,27,30] Vastus medialis plasty has primarily been investigated in comparative or randomized studies with findings demonstrating improvement in clinical outcomes measures and radiographic measures (including congruence angle, lateral patellofemoral angle, and lateral patellar displacement) in comparison to preoperative levels.[20,28,29] While limited, semitendinosus tenodesis has primarily been investigated in case series of small cohorts.[25,26] The reported results demonstrated high levels of continued instability (up to 82%) with 35% of patients requiring a subsequent procedure at a nearly 6-year follow-up.[26]

In terms of comparative or randomized controlled trials (RCTs), multiple studies have investigated outcomes between medial retinaculum plication and vastus medialis plasty. In an RCT, Zhao and colleagues[28] reported that on computed tomography (CT) examination that both groups resulted in deterioration of the correction of the patellar position over time, with the medial retinaculum plication no longer demonstrating improved patellar position in comparison to the presurgical position. In addition, the vastus medialis plasty demonstrated significant better clinical outcome measures at all time points versus medial retinaculum plication. They also reported lower dislocation rates versus plication (7.7% vs 17.9%, respectively), although this was not statistically significant. Two studies by another group found similarly significantly improved clinical outcome measures and CT measurements with vastus medialis plasty in comparison to medial retinaculum plication.[19,31] Ma and colleagues[20] also performed an RCT comparing vastus medialis plasty and MPFL reconstruction. They reported no significant differences between groups on CT measurements (congruence angle, patellar tilt angle, or patellar lateral shift), clinical outcome measures (Tegner or Kujala), or positive apprehension tests.[20]

Lastly, systematic reviews and meta-analyses have evaluated medial retinaculum plication and vastus medialis plasty. Lee and colleagues[17] performed a systematic review and meta-analysis and reported that patients with recurrent patellar instability had higher Lysholm and Kujala scores after MPFL reconstruction in comparison with medial soft tissue realignment surgery. Similar results were reported by Previtali and colleagues,[22] in a meta-analysis of medial soft tissue techniques and MPFL reconstruction. They reported similarly improved clinical outcomes (Lysholm and Kujala scores) after MPFL reconstruction in comparison to medial-based techniques. They also reported lower redislocation rates in MPFL reconstruction versus medial-based procedures (0.7% vs 2.9%, respectively), although this was not significant.[22] It should be noted that in contrast to Lee and colleagues,[17] Previtali and colleagues[22] only included studies that involved patients without untreated anatomic predisposing abnormalities.

Even in the absence of skeletal or constitutional risk factors for recurrent instability, the authors feel that there is no clear role for performing the above-described nonanatomic procedures. Anatomic MPFL repair may be considered in limited setting as detailed below.

MEDIAL PATELLOFEMORAL LIGAMENT REPAIR HAS A LIMITED ROLE IN THE ACUTE SETTING

An acute first-time dislocation must be considered as a distinct clinical entity from patients with recurrent instability. In these patients, we advocate the use of comprehensive history, clinical examination, and imaging to characterize the lesion, presence of associated injuries, and to identify risk factors for recurrence. MRI is recommended by a majority of specialist patellofemoral surgeons in this setting.[32] In the absence of surgical intervention, and particularly in the setting of recurrent instability episodes, the MPFL (and other medial structures) may heal with a degree of laxity and loss of function.

Historically, many have advocated for the nonoperative management of patients with a first-time dislocation. This has been supported by systematic reviews of clinical studies concluding that surgical treatment for first-time dislocation is not superior to conservative treatment in terms of clinical outcomes including the Kujala and Tegner scores and redislocation.[6,17] As such, nonoperative management for acute first-time patella dislocation remains the standard of care. However, current data have highlighted a potential role for operative management following acute dislocations in select patients. In 2018, The International Patellofemoral Study Group (IPSG) sought to achieve consensus on various aspects of the management of patella instability. In the acute setting, this group of experienced patellofemoral surgeons unanimously supported a role for concomitant surgery to address instability in patients with a first-time dislocation *with* an operative osteochondral fracture requiring fixation.[32]

Several authors have advocated for MPFL repair in this setting citing the below concerns with acute MPFL reconstruction. These include the risk of stiffness, requirement of an additional graft harvest, risks and costs associated with allograft use, and technical challenges of reconstruction. However, there are several critical prerequisites to considering this approach (**Box 1**). It is increasingly clear that MPFL repair is associated with unacceptably high failure rates in patients with established risk factors for recurrence—namely, patella alta, trochlear dysplasia, and an elevated TT-TG distance.[33–37] Overall, MPFL repairs that involve an avulsion from the femoral or patellar attachment with an otherwise intact ligament with good tissue quality appear to do best.[10,35] Multifocal or midsubstance tears are therefore considered relative contraindications to MPFL repair.[10,35] The soft tissue quality must also be sufficiently good to support repair.

Early studies demonstrated favorable results following acute medial soft tissue repair in the setting of patellar instability.[11,33,34,38,39] However, several trials have demonstrated no statistically significant difference between acute repair versus conservative treatments in terms of recurrent instability rates and outcome scores.[40,41] Others have found a higher failure rate following repair when contrasted to reconstruction despite some demonstrating similar outcome scores and return to sport.[39]

There are reports of good outcomes with improved patient-reported outcome scores in individuals managed acutely with MPFL repair. Camanho and colleagues[42] compared conservative treatment to acute MPFL repair in 33 patients and found that acute repair was associated with higher Kujala scores than conservative treatment with no recurrent instability. Ahmad and colleagues reported similar improvements with high levels of satisfaction and patient outcome scores following acute repair.[38] Pedowitz and colleagues followed a series of 41 patients managed surgically with MPFL repair at the time of addressing osteochondral defects. Though the technique of surgical repair varied within this series (9 open and 7 arthroscopic) and location of the tear was not uniform (7 patellar, 4 midsubstance, 2 multiple, 3 unknown), they found that MPFL repair did not reduce the rate of recurrent instability.[43] Christiansen and colleagues have showed no reduction in recurrence of instability following acute repair. However, all patients in their series underwent receiving femoral-based procedures and it is unclear whether midsubstance and patellar-based tears were present.[44] Askenberger and colleagues showed minimal difference in Kujala scores between operatively and nonoperatively treated patients despite significant differences in redislocation rates.[33]

Box 1
Prerequisites for MPFL repair in the acute setting

- Presence of osteochondral fragment requiring surgical intervention
- Single tear to MPFL in defined location
- Good tissue quality
- Absence of anatomic risk factors for recurrent instability (patella alta, increased TT-TG, increased q-angle, trochlear dysplasia)

Synthesis of the clinical literature is challenging given heterogeneity in patient, injury, underlying anatomic factors, and surgical factors. It is our interpretation that MPFL reconstruction remains the gold-standard procedure to perform concomitantly when addressing acute osteochondral lesions following an acute patella dislocation. However, MPFL repair can be considered when there is good tissue quality with a singular defined tear location and normal bony anatomy.

Surgical Technique for Medial Patellofemoral Ligament Repair in Acute Setting

A variety of both arthroscopic and open techniques have been described for medial soft tissue repair or medial patellofemoral ligament repair.[13,33,34,38,45,46] A diagnostic arthroscopy is first performed to evaluate and address concurrent intraarticular pathology. Once intra-articular pathology is addressed, patellar and femoral avulsions can be addressed through mini-open approaches. Patella avulsions can be addressed via a direct approach to the medial aspect of the patella, where the MPFL remnant can be found deep to the medial crural fascia and evaluated for its tissue quality and the feasibility of repair. If the intra-articular pathology needs to be addressed open, this plane can be exploited to facilitate a medial parapatellar arthrotomy. It is beneficial to identify the layers medially and the remnant MPFL tissue before completing a full arthrotomy to more readily facilitate repair. For femoral-based avulsions, a more medially based incision can be used overlying the adductor tubercle and the femoral insertion of the MPFL. If intra-articular pathology needs to be addressed open concurrently with a femoral avulsion, consideration can be given to intra-articular access through a lateral parapatellar arthrotomy or lengthening so as to not violate the native patellar MPFL attachment. Once the intraarticular pathology is addressed, anatomic repair can be performed advancing the tissue to the patellar or femoral origin and secured using suture anchor or screw fixation (**Fig. 1**). Following this, additional superficial soft tissue imbrication can be performed to aid in augmenting the acute repair.

MEDIAL PATELLOFEMORAL LIGAMENT REPAIR IN THE CHRONIC SETTING

In the setting of recurrent instability, it is the consensus among experts that surgical stabilization is indicated and this has become the standard of care.[47] In addition to the intrusive symptoms that can be associated with instability, recent articles have

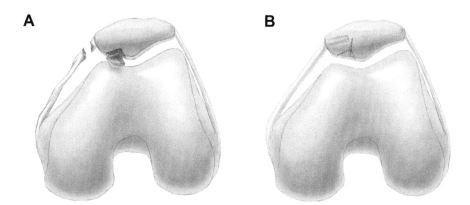

A   **B**

Fig. 1. Acute anatomic MPFL repair. (*A*) Axial image of clear injury to femoral or patella insertion of MPFL with intra-articular bony defect. (*B*) Axial image following anchor repair of MPFL and evidence of fixation of chondral fragment.

shown high rates of patellofemoral arthritis with nonoperative treatment of patellar instability. However, whether surgery can affect the progression to osteoarthritis is disputed.[48] The vast majority of surgeons in the IPFSG felt the need to reconstruct, rather than repair, the medial soft-tissue restraints (MPFL, medial quads tendon-femoral ligament) which is in line with recent literature suggesting up to 46% failure rate in MPFL repair with recurrent dislocations[13,44,49,50] compared with modern failure rates of 1% to 7% for MPFL reconstruction at short-term to midterm follow-up.[14,15] As such MPFL reconstruction patients with recurrent instability despite a comprehensive nonoperative patellar stabilization program remains the gold standard. Potential reasons for reduced efficacy of repair in the chronic setting may include chronic deficiency of the residual ligament with less strength and stiffness than those of the allograft tendon.

Prior studies have shown mixed outcomes after MPFL repair with recurrence rates ranging from 17% to 46% at 2 to 4 years of follow-up. Studies directly comparing repair versus reconstruction have mostly included patients with concomitant anatomic risk factors such as patella alta or tuberosity malalignment, which are known to influence MPFL biomechanics. Prevtali and colleagues[22] sought to address this issue by identifying studies that enabled more detailed analysis of these factors. They included 319 knees from 6 studies and reported no significant difference in rates of recurrent dislocation or minor complications at 2 to 5 yrs of follow-up between MPFL reconstruction and repair. However, they reported significant differences in Kujala and Lysholm scores favoring reconstruction in both short-term and long-term follow-up. They reported on subgroup analyses isolating reconstruction techniques with a range of predisposing factors, with all functional outcomes significantly favoring MPFL reconstruction over repair with the exception of the Tegner score.

There is growing evidence supporting the role of MPFL reconstruction over repair in the setting of recurrent patella instability. Bitar and colleagues[51,52] reported superior outcomes with MPFL reconstruction over MPFL repair. Puzzitiello and colleagues[39] collected outcomes of 32 reconstructions and 19 repairs with a 59.7-month follow-up period finding that MPFL reconstruction outperformed repair. The surgical techniques in this study varied with a range of methods of patella and femur fixation MPFL reconstructions as well as different MPFL repair techniques. Although the lack of consistency in surgical techniques in this and other studies is a limitation, overall it appears that MPFL repair is less reliable than MPFL reconstruction.

When interpreting the data, it is important to recognize that patient-reported outcome measures and rates of recurrent instability do not always correlate. Puzzitiello and colleagues[39] reported a failure rate after isolated MPFL repair that was 6-fold higher than following isolated MPFL reconstruction at a minimum follow-up of 2 years (36.9% vs 6.3%), despite finding no significant difference in Kujala scores between groups. Similarly, Sherman and colleagues[53] reported a recurrent instability rate at 6 months of 0% (0 of 29 cases) following MPFL reconstruction and 33.3% (8 of 24) following repair, despite similar PROMS in a series of patients younger than 18 years. Several recent publications have shown comparable outcomes when assessing MPFL repair or MPFL reconstruction alone. Studies by Camp and colleagues[13] and Arendt and colleagues[49] reported similarly high rates of recurrent instability (28% and 46%, respectively) following isolated MPFL repair at a minimum of 2 years. A recent systematic review by Schneider and colleagues[54] reported a pooled risk of recurrent instability of 1.2% following MPFL reconstruction.

Despite this, proponents of MPFL repair argue that this strategy offers significant benefits over reconstruction including being technically easier with lower risks of morbidity, while reconstruction graft mal-positioning or over-tensioning, as well as the risk of patella fracture, can occur with reconstruction. While accepting that MPFL reconstruction remains the most appropriate operative strategy in the majority of cases, they intimate that there may be a limited role for MPFL repair in a limited number of well-defined settings. Indeed, Dragoo and colleagues[35] have shown some excellent outcomes with repair in the setting of a TT-TG distance of under 2 cm with the avulsion occurring from either the patellar the femur. However, this study again emphasizes the limited scope of repair, which is best supported only in the setting of bony avulsions from the patella or femur in the absence of concurrent anomalous bony anatomy predisposing to recurrence.

i. Patulous MPFL in the Absence of Risk Factors

In patients with recurrent instability, who have developed an expanded or patulous MPFL but in whom the tissue quality remains good there may be a role for anatomic repair through restoration of the native working length (**Fig. 2**). In these patients, the working length and function of the MPFL as a check-rein to lateral patella translation is restored. In these patients, the MPFL is detached from the patella and the lateral edge excised back to its working length before reattachment to the patella using anchors (see **Fig. 2; Fig. 3**).

ii. Repairs when Alignment is Being Corrected Concomitantly

To date, the authors are not aware of studies comparing outcomes of MPFL repair and reconstruction when performed as part of combined procedures to address underlying bony abnormalities such as with tibial tubercle osteotomies. In this setting, key drivers of instability are being addressed and the repair procedure could be considered analogous to soft tissue balancing, taking up the resting length of the redundant MPFL. Further data in these settings is required to establish the role of MPFL repair in this setting.

CHALLENGES OF INTERPRETING LITERATURE IN THE SETTING OF MEDIAL PATELLOFEMORAL LIGAMENT REPAIR

There are several challenges that limit our ability to interpret existing data and to establish the most effective strategies to address medial soft tissue dysfunction. The numerous permutations of morphologic risk factors in patients with patellar

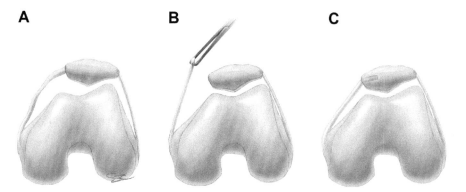

Fig. 2. Anatomic repair for patulous but intact MPFL. (*A*) Axial image showing patulous MPFL. (*B*) Axial image showing patulous MPFL lifted off patella and held with Alice clamp. (*C*) Axial image showing completed repair.

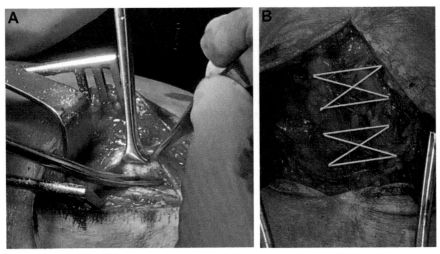

Fig. 3. Clinical photographs of anatomic repair for patulous MPFL. (*A*) Dissection between layers of the medial knee to identify and isolate the patulous MPFL. (*B*) Superficial soft tissue imbrication with "X-box" configuration of sutures can be performed to augment the repair.

instability have made it difficult to determine the clinical benefits of one procedure over another, even in larger series and trials. Heterogeneity between surgical techniques also negates direct comparison between procedures. In certain studies, the term "MPFL repair" is used to described plication, reefing, augmentation, imbrication, and medial soft tissue plasty.[22] Heterogeneity in MPFL reconstruction techniques is also problematic. Several studies and systematic reviews of studies do not differentiate between acute and chronic, despite these representing very different clinical entities.[50]

SUMMARY

The most appropriate surgical strategy to address MPFL deficiency following acute and recurrent patella instability continues to be the subject of considerable debate. Overall, when surgery is indicated, existing data would support a role for MPFL reconstruction and this remains the gold-standard procedure for addressing soft tissue deficiency in the absence of anatomic risk factors for recurrence. However, MPFL repair has many theoretic advantages over MPFL reconstruction and nonanatomical approaches but its widespread use has not been supported by recent clinical literature. Despite this, MPFL repair may continue to have a limited role in the setting of acute and chronic surgical stabilization. Current understanding on the role of MPFL repair is challenging because of a lack of high-level evidence as well as numerous complex variables influencing decision making. High-quality, multicenter RCTs, particularly comparing MPFL repair with MPFL reconstruction while controlling for underlying risk factors, are needed.

REFERENCES

1. Fithian DC, Paxton EW, Stone ML, et al. Epidemiology and natural history of acute patellar dislocation. Am J Sports Med 2004;32(5):1114–21.
2. Nietosvaara Y, Aalto K, Kallio PE. Acute patellar dislocation in children: incidence and associated osteochondral fractures. J Pediatr Orthop 1994;14(4):513–5.

3. Lewallen L, McIntosh A, Dahm D. First-time patellofemoral dislocation: risk factors for recurrent instability. J Knee Surg 2015;28(4):303–9.

4. Lewallen LW, McIntosh AL, Dahm DL. Predictors of recurrent instability after acute patellofemoral dislocation in pediatric and adolescent patients. Am J Sports Med 2013;41(3):575–81.

5. Nwachukwu BU, So C, Schairer WW, et al. Surgical versus conservative management of acute patellar dislocation in children and adolescents: a systematic review. Knee Surg Sports Traumatol Arthrosc 2016;24(3):760–7.

6. Palmu S, Kallio PE, Donell ST, et al. Acute patellar dislocation in children and adolescents: a randomized clinical trial. J Bone Joint Surg Am 2008;90(3):463–70.

7. Weber AE, Nathani A, Dines JS, et al. An algorithmic approach to the management of recurrent lateral patellar dislocation. J Bone Joint Surg Am 2016;98(5): 417–27.

8. Conlan T, Garth WP Jr, Lemons JE. Evaluation of the medial soft-tissue restraints of the extensor mechanism of the knee. J Bone Joint Surg Am. 1993;75(5): 682–93.

9. Askenberger M, Arendt EA, Ekström W, et al. Medial patellofemoral ligament injuries in children with first-time lateral patellar dislocations: a magnetic resonance imaging and arthroscopic study. Am J Sports Med 2016;44(1):152–8.

10. Duchman KR, Bollier MJ. The role of medial patellofemoral ligament repair and imbrication. Am J Orthop (Belle Mead NJ) 2017;46(2):87–91.

11. Sallay PI, Poggi J, Speer KP, et al. Acute dislocation of the patella. A correlative pathoanatomic study. Am J Sports Med 1996;24(1):52–60.

12. Zhang GY, Zheng L, Shi H, et al. Injury patterns of medial patellofemoral ligament after acute lateral patellar dislocation in children: correlation analysis with anatomical variants and articular cartilage lesion of the patella. Eur Radiol 2017;27(3):1322–30.

13. Camp CL, Krych AJ, Dahm DL, et al. Medial patellofemoral ligament repair for recurrent patellar dislocation. Am J Sports Med 2010;38(11):2248–54.

14. Balcarek P, Rehn S, Howells NR, et al. Results of medial patellofemoral ligament reconstruction compared with trochleoplasty plus individual extensor apparatus balancing in patellar instability caused by severe trochlear dysplasia: a systematic review and meta-analysis. Knee Surg Sports Traumatol Arthrosc 2017;25(12): 3869–77.

15. Stephen JM, Lumpaopong P, Deehan DJ, et al. The medial patellofemoral ligament: location of femoral attachment and length change patterns resulting from anatomic and nonanatomic attachments. Am J Sports Med 2012;40(8):1871–9.

16. Barkatali BM, Lea M, Aster A, et al. Arthroscopic medial capsular plication using the suture anchor technique. Knee Surg Sports Traumatol Arthrosc 2014;22(10): 2513–7.

17. Lee DY, Park YJ, Song SY, et al. Which technique is better for treating patellar dislocation? a systematic review and meta-analysis. Arthroscopy 2018;34(11): 3082–93, e3081.

18. Lee JJ, Lee SJ, Won YG, et al. Lateral release and medial plication for recurrent patella dislocation. Knee Surg Sports Traumatol Arthrosc 2012;20(12):2438–44.

19. Ma LF, Wang CH, Chen BC, et al. Medial patellar retinaculum plasty versus medial capsule reefing for patellar dislocation in children and adolescents. Arch Orthop Trauma Surg 2012;132(12):1773–80.

20. Ma LF, Wang F, Chen BC, et al. Medial retinaculum plasty versus medial patellofemoral ligament reconstruction for recurrent patellar instability in adults: a randomized controlled trial. Arthroscopy 2013;29(5):891–7.

21. Miller JR, Adamson GJ, Pink MM, et al. Arthroscopically assisted medial reefing without routine lateral release for patellar instability. Am J Sports Med 2007;35(4): 622–9.

22. Previtali D, Milev SR, Pagliazzi G, et al. Recurrent patellar dislocations without un-treated predisposing factors: medial patellofemoral ligament reconstruction versus other medial soft-tissue surgical techniques-a meta-analysis. Arthroscopy 2020;36(6):1725–34.

23. Song JG, Kang SB, Oh SH, et al. Medial soft-tissue realignment versus medial patellofemoral ligament reconstruction for recurrent patellar dislocation: system-atic review. Arthroscopy 2016;32(3):507–16.

24. Galeazzi R. New applications of muscle and tendon transplant. Arch Di Ortop Mi-lano 1922;315–23.

25. Aulisa AG, Falciglia F, Giordano M, et al. Galeazzi's modified technique for recur-rent patella dislocation in skeletally immature patients. J Orthop Sci 2012;17(2): 148–55.

26. Grannatt K, Heyworth BE, Ogunwole O, et al. Galeazzi semitendinosus tenodesis for patellofemoral instability in skeletally immature patients. J Pediatr Orthop 2012;32(6):621–5.

27. Halbrecht JL. Arthroscopic patella realignment: an all-inside technique. Arthros-copy 2001;17(9):940–5.

28. Zhao J, Huangfu X, He Y. The role of medial retinaculum plication versus medial patellofemoral ligament reconstruction in combined procedures for recurrent patellar instability in adults. Am J Sports Med 2012;40(6):1355–64.

29. James AW, Zara JN, Corselli M, et al. An abundant perivascular source of stem cells for bone tissue engineering. Stem Cells Transl Med 2012;1(9):673–84.

30. Nam EK, Karzel RP. Mini-open medial reefing and arthroscopic lateral release for the treatment of recurrent patellar dislocation: a medium-term follow-up. Am J Sports Med 2005;33(2):220–30.

31. Ma LF, Wang F, Chen BC, et al. Medial patellar retinaculum plasty versus medial capsule reefing for patellar subluxation in adult. Orthop Surg 2012;4(2):83–8.

32. Liu JN, Steinhaus ME, Kalbian IL, et al. Patellar instability management: a survey of the international patellofemoral study group. Am J Sports Med 2018;46(13): 3299–306.

33. Askenberger M, Bengtsson Mostrom E, Ekstrom W, et al. Operative repair of medial patellofemoral ligament injury versus knee brace in children with an acute first-time traumatic patellar dislocation: a randomized controlled trial. Am J Sports Med 2018;46(10):2328–40.

34. Cerciello S, Lustig S, Costanzo G, et al. Medial retinaculum reefing for the treat-ment for patellar instability. Knee Surg Sports Traumatol Arthrosc 2014;22(10): 2505–12.

35. Dragoo JL, Nguyen M, Gatewood CT, et al. Medial patellofemoral ligament repair versus reconstruction for recurrent patellar instability: two-year results of an algorithm-based approach. Orthop J Sports Med 2017;5(3). 2325967116689465.

36. Hevesi M, Heidenreich MJ, Camp CL, et al. The recurrent instability of the patella score: a statistically based model for prediction of long-term recurrence risk after first-time dislocation. Arthroscopy 2019;35(2):537–43.

37. Rund JM, Hinckel BB, Sherman SL. Acute patellofemoral dislocation: controver-sial decision-making. Curr Rev Musculoskelet Med 2021;14(1):82–7.

38. Ahmad CS, Shubin Stein BE, Matuz D, et al. Immediate surgical repair of the medial patellar stabilizers for acute patellar dislocation. A review of eight cases. Am J Sports Med 2000;28(6):804–10.

39. Puzzitiello RN, Waterman B, Agarwalla A, et al. Primary medial patellofemoral ligament repair versus reconstruction: rates and risk factors for instability recurrence in a young, active patient population. Arthroscopy 2019;35(10):2909–15.
40. Migliorini F, Driessen A, Quack V, et al. Surgical versus conservative treatment for first patellofemoral dislocations: a meta-analysis of clinical trials. Eur J Orthop Surg Traumatol 2020;30(5):771–80.
41. Tian G, Yang G, Zuo L, et al. Conservative versus repair of medial patellofemoral ligament for the treatment of patients with acute primary patellar dislocations: a systematic review and meta-analysis. J Orthop Surg (Hong Kong) 2020;28(2). 2309499020932375.
42. Camanho GL, Viegas Ade C, Bitar AC, et al. Conservative versus surgical treatment for repair of the medial patellofemoral ligament in acute dislocations of the patella. Arthroscopy 2009;25(6):620–5.
43. Pedowitz JM, Edmonds EW, Chambers HG, et al. Recurrence of patellar instability in adolescents undergoing surgery for osteochondral defects without concomitant ligament reconstruction. Am J Sports Med 2019;47(1):66–70.
44. Christiansen SE, Jakobsen BW, Lund B, et al. Isolated repair of the medial patellofemoral ligament in primary dislocation of the patella: a prospective randomized study. Arthroscopy 2008;24(8):881–7.
45. Sillanpaa PJ, Maenpaa HM, Mattila VM, et al. Arthroscopic surgery for primary traumatic patellar dislocation: a prospective, nonrandomized study comparing patients treated with and without acute arthroscopic stabilization with a median 7-year follow-up. Am J Sports Med 2008;36(12):2301–9.
46. Sillanpaa PJ, Salonen E, Pihlajamaki H, et al. Medial patellofemoral ligament avulsion injury at the patella: classification and clinical outcome. Knee Surg Sports Traumatol Arthrosc 2014;22(10):2414–8.
47. Strickland SM. Editorial commentary: medial patellofemoral ligament repair versus reconstruction: still a question or a clear winner? Arthroscopy 2019; 35(10):2916–7.
48. Sanders TL, Pareek A, Johnson NR, et al. Patellofemoral arthritis after lateral patellar dislocation: a matched population-based analysis. Am J Sports Med 2017;45(5):1012–7.
49. Arendt EA, Moeller A, Agel J. Clinical outcomes of medial patellofemoral ligament repair in recurrent (chronic) lateral patella dislocations. Knee Surg Sports Traumatol Arthrosc 2011;19(11):1909–14.
50. Matic GT, Magnussen RA, Kolovich GP, et al. Return to activity after medial patellofemoral ligament repair or reconstruction. Arthroscopy 2014;30(8):1018–25.
51. Bitar AC, D'Elia CO, Demange MK, et al. Randomized prospective study on traumatic patellar dislocation: conservative treatment versus reconstruction of the medial patellofemoral ligament using the patellar tendon, with a minimum of two years of follow-up. Rev Bras Ortop 2011;46(6):675–83.
52. Bitar AC, Demange MK, D'Elia CO, et al. Traumatic patellar dislocation: nonoperative treatment compared with MPFL reconstruction using patellar tendon. Am J Sports Med 2012;40(1):114–22.
53. Sherman SL, Geeslin DW, Hogan DW, et al. Comparison of MPFL repair versus MPFL reconstruction for refractory patella instability in patients under 18 years old. Orthop J Sports Med 2020. https://doi.org/10.1177/2325967120S00189.
54. Schneider DK, Grawe B, Magnussen RA, et al. Outcomes after isolated medial patellofemoral ligament reconstruction for the treatment of recurrent lateral patellar dislocations: a systematic review and meta-analysis. Am J Sports Med 2016;44(11):2993–3005.

The Lateral Side
When and How to Release, Lengthen, and Reconstruct

Navya Dandu, BS, Nicholas A. Trasolini, MD,
Steven F. DeFroda, MD, Reem Y. Darwish, BS,
Adam B. Yanke, MD, PhD*

KEYWORDS

- Lateral retinaculum • Medial instability • LPFL • Reconstruction • Lengthening
- Release

KEY POINTS

- The lateral patellofemoral complex has an important role in both lateral and medial patellar displacement.
- Lateral lengthening is recommended over lateral release owing to the high incidence of iatrogenic medial instability after release.
- Lateral reconstruction is a viable option for the treatment of iatrogenic medial instability.

INTRODUCTION

Proper patellar tracking throughout flexion relies on the alignment and balance of several soft tissues and osseus stabilizers.[1] The medial patellofemoral complex and the lateral patellofemoral complex (LPFC) are the primary static stabilizers in early flexion before engagement with the trochlea. Abnormalities of the lateral structures, ranging from tightness to laxity, can be addressed surgically in the way of lateral retinacular lengthening or lateral patellofemoral ligament (LPFL) reconstruction.[2] Historically, lateral retinacular release has been performed as a concomitant procedure in the setting of patellar instability or patellofemoral pain. However, owing to the high risk of iatrogenic medial instability, and the paradoxic increase of lateral translation, lengthening is now recommended in place of a full release when possible. The

ABY receives research support from Arthrex, Inc, Vericel, and Organogenesis. Dr. Yanke is a paid consultant for CONMED Linvatec, JRF Ortho, and Olympus and an unpaid consultant for PatientIQ, Smith & Nephew, and Sparta Biomedical. He has stock or stock options in PatientIQ.
N. Dandu, N.A. Trasolini, S.F. DeFroda, and R.Y. Darwish have nothing to disclose.
Rush University Medical Center, 1611 West Harrison Street, Suite 300, Chicago, IL 60612, USA
* Corresponding author.
E-mail address: Adam.yanke@rushortho.com

objective of this article is to review the relevant presentation, clinical examination, anatomy, and surgical treatment options for lateral patellofemoral dysfunction.

HISTORY AND PRESENTATION

Patients with patellofemoral soft tissue imbalance can frequently present with arthritis, lateral compression syndrome, anterior knee pain, and patellar instability.[3,4] Patients with a history of prior lateral retinacular release can present with iatrogenic medial instability, although they may not always describe the patella dislocating medially.[5] Typically, it is helpful to use a patellar stabilizing brace with the mechanism reversed to resist medial displacement. This technique should feel more comfortable to patients than resisting lateral displacement and helps to confirm the diagnosis of medial instability. Compression syndrome frequently presents progressively, classically aggravated by prolonged flexion. Pain is typically worsened with stairs, with descending stairs being more symptomatic than climbing stairs. Swelling may present as stiffness after activity and it is typically indicative of arthritis or chondral damage.

PHYSICAL EXAMINATION

The physical examination can help to further evaluate the integrity of the lateral retinaculum on initial presentation. Specifically, a patellar translation (glide) test can establish laxity or tightness based on medial translation, with more than 3 quadrants or less than 1 quadrant indicating those pathologies respectively (**Fig. 1**A).[2] Similarly, a medial patellar tilt of 15° to 20° asymmetry compared with the contralateral side or more than 45° can indicate lateral laxity, and this can range up to 90° in the setting of prior

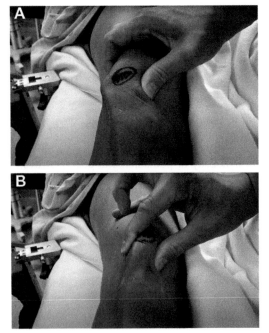

Fig. 1. Examination under anesthesia in a patient with a prior lateral release demonstrates (A) a fully dislocatable patella with 4 quadrants of lateral translation and (B) lateral eversion of the patella to almost 90°.

lateral release (**Fig. 1**B).[2] Patients with medial instability will also typically notice apprehension with medial patellar glide that feels similar to their complaints of apprehension.

After assessment of soft tissues, the following measures of rotational profile and lower limb alignment should be considered as potential contributions to patellar maltracking:

- Q-angle[6]
- Clinical coronal alignment
- Femoral anteversion[7]

Other physical examination findings classically associated with patellar instability, such as the J-sign and patellar apprehension, may indicate the presence of other underlying pathoanatomic factors that need to be confirmed with imaging, such as trochlear dysplasia.[6,8] The presence of these factors should be taken into consideration when formulating a surgical plan in the setting of instability. Patellofemoral grind may result in pain and crepitus, with crepitus indicating underlying chondral damage. The amount of crepitation in the patellofemoral joint can be accentuated with a single leg squat.

IMAGING

In the setting of lateral patellar instability with excessive lateral tilt, associated pathoanatomic factors should be investigated before assuming a retinacular origin. On radiographic merchant views, the following should be evaluated:

- Lateral patellofemoral angle: Formed by a line tangent to medial and lateral femoral condyles and a line tangent to the lateral patellar facet. An angle of less than 11° is cited as an abnormal lateral contracture.[9]
- Patellofemoral index: The ratio of the medial and lateral patellofemoral joint spaces, which is normally less than 1.6, with an increased ratio (decreased lateral space) indicating lateral contracture.[10]
- Coronal alignment: Distal femoral valgus[11] mechanical axis[7]

On computed tomography scans and MRI, the following points should be evaluated:

- Lateral retinacular redundancy: The appearance of the retinacular structure in the context of patellar positioning can provide insight into its contribution. In the setting of excessive tilt, if the retinaculum is redundant then other causes of tilt should be explored. Prior lateral release can also be observed if the patient is unable to provide detailed surgical history (**Fig. 2**).[2]
- Trochlear dysplasia: Can lead to patellar tilt. Correction of trochlear dysplasia is not necessary for the efficacy of isolated lateral procedures.[12]
- Tibial tubercle–trochlear groove distance: An increased distance (15–20 mm) indicates a lateral vector on the extensor mechanism. Ratios can also be used to standardize the measurement to the patient's size.[13,14]
- Patellar tendon–lateral trochlear ridge distance: More novel measures of extensor mechanism alignment taking into consideration the alignment of the patellar tendon within the groove.[15]

ANATOMY AND FUNCTION
Lateral Patellofemoral Ligament Anatomy

Although the MPFL and medial patellofemoral complex has been well-studied, interest in the LPFL has also been emerging, with less robust research into the stability of the

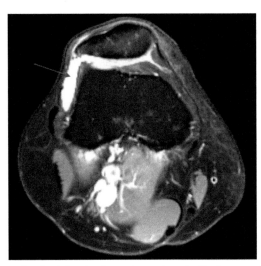

Fig. 2. MRI imaging of prior lateral release (arrow) and effusion associated with patellar instability.

LPFC.[16–22] The LPFL was first described by Kaplan, who defined the anatomy of the lateral side of the knee, and identified what was termed the "lateral epicondylar ligament," which was identified at the level of the deep transverse retinaculum.[21] This work was further confirmed by Fulkerson and colleagues,[20] and this structure was eventually renamed the LPFL by Reider and colleagues[23] in 1981 in a study in which a dissection of 48 knees was performed. Interestingly, the authors found that the width of the LPFL most correlated with the overall shape of the ligament.

An in-depth anatomic study in 2009 by Waligora and colleagues[24] described the anatomy of the extensor mechanism of the knee and found that the MPFL was far more common than the LPFL, and was more robust when both were present. In actuality, the authors only were able to describe an LPFL in 1 of 18 cadaveric specimens.[24] The authors did note, however, that their specimens were preserved in formalin, which likely altered the structure of the ligament making it difficult to isolate from the rest of the lateral capsular structures.[24] More recent studies have sought to define the true origin, insertion, and anatomic characteristics of the LPFL. Capkin and colleagues[19] recently reported their results of anatomic dissection of the LPFL on embalmed, human cadaveric knees. They described the anatomic origin of the ligament on the femur by dividing the lateral condyle into thirds in the vertical and sagittal plane, finding that the LPFL originated from the central section of the lateral condyle in both the vertical and sagittal planes, in a majority of the knees.[19] The authors did not, however, report on the patellar insertion. A 2017 study by Shah and colleagues[17] more clearly defined the anatomy of the LPFL. In this study, 10 fresh frozen cadavers were dissected and the LPFL patellar and femoral insertions were defined with respect to the superior–inferior axis of the lateral patella, and lateral epicondyle respectively. On average, the LPFL originated 2.6 cm distal and 10.8 mm anterior to the lateral epicondyle, with an average absolute distance of 14.5 mm from the epicondyle. The patellar insertion was found to be in the middle third of the articular surface, with an average width of 14.3 mm corresponding with 45% the articular surface height (range, 23.7%–58.4%).[17] The width at the femoral insertion averaged 11.7 mm. Of note, although the femoral anatomy was somewhat variable, 9 of 10 specimens had femoral attachments that were anterior to the epicondyle, whereas 7 of 10 were distal, demonstrating relative consistency as to its femoral insertion.[17] A similar study by Navarro and colleagues[22] including 20 fresh cadaveric knees found a similar average ligament width of 16.05 mm, but did not define patellar or femoral attachments.

The function of the LPFL with regard to patellar positioning has also been studied. Vieira and colleagues[25] first defined the LPFL and determined it to be a lateral capsular thickening measuring 1.3 cm in width. The authors then sectioned the ligament and found that the patella displaced medially, demonstrating the structure's importance in protecting the patella against medial instability. Unfortunately, unlike the MPFL and medial patellofemoral complex, the role of the LPFL in dynamic patellar tracking is less well-understood currently, necessitating further biomechanical studies in this area.[26,27]

Lateral Patellofemoral Ligament Biomechanics

Despite relatively limited attention to the LPFL compared with the MPFL, it is well-accepted that the LPFL plays an important role in the prevention of lateral patellar instability, in addition to providing the main restraint to medial patellar instability. Christian and colleagues[27] found that in the setting of MPFL sectioning, the addition of a lateral release of the LPFL actually increased lateral patellar translation, indicated that the LPFL and lateral capsule play a key role lateral patellar stability as well as being the primary medial stabilizer of the patella. Unfortunately, there are limited studies examining the biomechanical properties of the native LPFL. One study by DeFroda and colleagues[18] harvested 10 LPFL specimens with a bone plug from both the patellar and femoral side for ease of potting and biomechanical testing. The study aimed to determine if the anatomic properties of the ligament (midsubstance width, femoral insertion width, patellar width) influenced load to failure, as well as the most common mode of failure of the ligament. A mean load to failure of 90 N was reported, with 9 of 10 of the specimens failing at the midsubstance during load to failure testing. Additionally, it was found that the midsubstance width most correlated with overall load to failure; however, it did not reach statistical significance ($P = .09$).[18] The authors concluded that ultimately more studies are needed to further classify the biomechanics of the LPFL during dynamic testing and in the clinical setting of reconstruction.

It is believed that the biomechanical contributions of the LPFL and lateral capsule as a whole are most clinically significant with the knee in full extension. In extension, the patella is less constrained owing to the lack of engagement within the trochlea, even in patients with normal trochlear anatomy. However, it is worth noting that in extension the lateral trochlea is typically more prominent than the medial trochlea, allowing for additional bony restraint. The role that the lateral soft tissue stabilizers play in maintaining patellar stability at varying degrees of flexion and extension has been studied previously. Medial stability in an intact loaded knee has been shown to increase progressively from a mean of 78 N at 0° to 171 N at 90° of flexion during patellar engagement within the trochlea.[28] It is believed that the lateral capsule and its thickenings, of which the LPFL is the main contributor, play the most substantial role in stability at full extension, whereas the larger iliotibial band–patellar band is the primary stabilizer during flexion and trochlear engagement. Ghosh and colleagues[29] have shown the transverse iliotibial band–patellar band to be in a relaxed state when the knee is extended with significant tightening in flexion. A study by Merican and colleagues[28] supports this concept, showing that, upon releasing the iliotibial band–patellar band, patellar stability is significantly reduced at 30° to 90° of knee flexion. Conversely at 0° and

20° of flexion, the largest loss of stability is seen after LPFL/capsular release, with a decrease in medial stability of 13 ± 9 N, or 16% compared with the intact knee.[28]

SURGICAL TECHNIQUES
Lateral Release

Release of the lateral patellofemoral retinaculum was first described by Pollard[30] in 1891 in a case report of surgical treatment for flexion instability of the patella. Historical indications for lateral release have included lateral patellar instability,[31] patellofemoral pain of unknown origin refractory to conservative management,[32] patellofemoral pain with lateral patellar tilt (patellar compression syndrome),[33,34] patellar tracking correction after total knee arthroplasty in valgus knees,[35] and as an adjunct to distal realignment procedures.[36]

The current indications for lateral release have narrowed significantly. This change is due in part to inconsistent results of lateral release for both patellofemoral pain and patellar instability. In their review of lateral release for patellofemoral instability, Lattermann and colleagues[36] found that only 63.5% patient satisfaction at a minimum of 4 years of follow-up. Similarly, Panni and colleagues reported only 70% satisfaction after lateral release for patellofemoral pain at the long-term follow-up.[37] Additionally, reports of iatrogenic medial patellar instability after excessive lateral release have highlighted the morbidity of this procedure.[38] A consensus statement by the International Patellofemoral Study Group stated with 89% agreement that an isolated lateral release is never appropriate in the treatment of patellar instability.[39] However, some modern indications for lateral release remain. The authors' indications for lateral release include severe patella alta requiring distalization and distal translation of the lateral retinaculum, severe valgus deformity with lateral retinacular contracture that cannot be overcome with lateral lengthening alone, severe arthrofibrosis with decreased patellar mobility, and maltracking in the setting of total knee arthroplasty.

Lateral release can be performed through either a lateral parapatellar incision[40] or arthroscopically.[33,41] Open procedures allow for a more calculated release owing to direct visualization of the retinacular layer and vastus lateralis obliquus muscle, which should be preserved to decrease the risk of iatrogenic medial instability.[42,43] Additionally, the joint capsule can be preserved to prevent synovial fluid egress. Arthroscopic lateral release is less invasive superficially, but requires the release of the capsular layer as the retinaculum is incised from deep to superficial. In both cases, there is a risk of hemarthrosis or hematoma owing to the proximity of the lateral genicular arteries.[44] A randomized trial of 80 patients comparing the arthroscopic and open lateral release for lateral patellar compression syndrome found that arthroscopic release resulted in improved Lysholm scores and less iatrogenic medial instability.[45] In the authors' practice, arthroscopic lateral release is less often performed because the most common concomitant procedures (alta correction, valgus correction, or knee arthroplasty) necessitate an open approach.

Lateral Lengthening

Lengthening of the lateral patellofemoral retinaculum has become the preferred technique for the correction of pathologic lateral retinacular contracture. This technique was initially described by Larson and Slocum for the treatment of lateral patellar compression syndrome. In their technique, an open lateral incision was created down to the level of the lateral patellofemoral retinaculum.[46,47] The transverse fibers of the retinaculum were transected, and deep and superficial layers were developed. An arthrotomy was created to evaluate the joint surfaces, and then closed to prevent synovial fluid egress. The anterior edge of the deep retinacular layer and the posterior edge of the superficial layer were sutured to effectively lengthen the retinacular tissue.[48]

Modern techniques of lateral retinacular lengthening are largely unchanged from the original descriptions. Care is taken to isolate distinct superficial and deep layers of the retinacular tissue. The layers are divided in a step cut to allow for a calibrated amount of lengthening.[49] This step cut, or z-lengthening, begins with the superficial layer being divided 1 cm from the lateral patellar border.[50] The deep retinacular layer is then developed and transected 1 to 3 cm posterior to the division in the superficial retinacular layer. The superficial layer is then sutured to the deep layer to increase the retinacular length (**Fig. 3**). The maximum lengthening that can be achieved is determined by the distance from the superficial retinacular incision to the confluence of the anterior border of the iliotibial band and posterior border of the vastus lateralis fascia.[50] This location approximates the origin of the LPFL complex.[51] An arthrotomy is avoided in modern techniques because a concurrent arthroscopy is performed to evaluate the intra-articular structures.

Lateral lengthening is performed most commonly in conjunction with distal realignment or medial patellofemoral complex reconstruction. In these scenarios, the lateral retinaculum is released in a step cut calibrated to the planned length correction. A distal realignment and/or medial reconstruction is then performed and the lateral retinaculum is closed at the desired length at the conclusion of the procedure.[49,52] In some cases, the required correction is too large to be achieved with a step cut and a lateral release with a LPFL reconstruction or patch augmentation is required.[50]

Rehabilitation protocols are determined in large part by concurrent procedures and the addition of a lateral lengthening does not change the postoperative restrictions or physical therapy protocol in those scenarios. In the case of an isolated lateral lengthening, the knee is placed into a hinged brace that is locked in extension during weight-bearing until protective quadriceps strength returns. Motion is unrestricted when the patient is not bearing weight.

Outcomes of Lateral Lengthening Versus Lateral Release

Several trials have compared lateral lengthening to lateral release. A prospective, randomized comparison of 86 patients undergoing arthroscopic lateral release versus open lateral lengthening found improved Lysholm scores with the open lateral

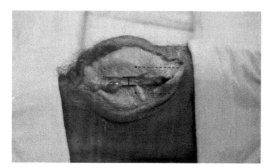

Fig. 3. Cadaveric demonstration of a lateral lengthening approach. An incision is made in the superficial retinacular layer (*blue arrows*) more anterior to the incision made in the deep layer (*white arrow*). The distance between these incisions is equal to the amount of lengthening achieved (*black bracket*).

lengthening with no difference in range of motion, thigh circumference, or isokinetic quadriceps strength at a mean of 46 months of follow-up.[53] Another comparison of 28 patients randomized to open lateral release or open lateral lengthening found that 5 of 14 releases and 0 of 14 lengthenings resulted in iatrogenic medial instability.[54] In this study, lateral release also resulted in greater quadriceps atrophy and worse Kujala scores at minimum of 2 years of follow-up. It should be noted that the lateral release performed in this study was more aggressive than original descriptions of that technique.[55] Finally, a prospective study of 59 patients undergoing lateral release versus lateral retinaculum plasty (a lateral lengthening procedure) at the time of medial patellofemoral ligament reconstruction found worse Kujala scores and more instability on medial patellar glide test in the lateral release cohort at a minimum of 2 years of follow-up.

Lateral Patellofemoral Ligament Reconstruction

LPFL reconstruction was developed to address medial iatrogenic instability after lateral release.[38,56] There are reports of medial patellar instability without a prior lateral release, but these make up an extremely rare group, with only 6 total cases identified by members of the International Patellofemoral Study Group.[57] For both iatrogenic and noniatrogenic medial patellar instability, the treatment involves reconstruction of the lateral retinacular restraint.

The first graft-based reconstruction was described by Teitge[56] using a bone–quadriceps tendon autograft to create a LPFL. The bone plug of the graft was docked into the femur at the lateral epicondyle and the soft tissue end was passed transversely through a patellar bone tunnel. Saper and colleagues have described 2 techniques for LPFL reconstruction.[58,59] In the first, the central one-third of the quadriceps tendon is divided proximally, rotated laterally, and fixed to the femur at the lateral epicondyle.[58] In the second, a gracilis allograft tendon is looped through the proximal lateral patellar periosteum and then secured to the femur at the LPFL origin using an interference screw.[59] Another technique has described using a suture button to secure a looped end of a free graft to the femur, with the free ends of the graft secured at an appropriate length to the lateral and anterior patellar periosteum.[60] Sawyer and colleagues reported a lateral patellotibial reconstruction technique using patellar tendon and iliotibial band autograft, which was a modification of a method initially described by Hughston in 1996.[61,62] The lateral 8 mm of the patellar tendon is removed from the tibial tubercle, but remains attached to the patella; similarly, the anterior 8 mm of the iliotibial band is released proximally and remains attached to Gerdy's tubercle. The 2 grafts are then sutured together, essentially tethering the lateral border of the patella to Gerdy's tubercle at the appropriate length to prevent medial patellar subluxation without capturing the knee. Although there are various techniques described in the literature, all follow the basic principles of ligament reconstruction as outlined by Teitge and Spak, including the selection of a sufficiently strong graft, isometric graft placement, adequate fixation, correct tension, and no condylar rubbing or bony impingement.[56]

The authors' preferred technique for LPFL reconstruction uses a free hamstring allograft and an all soft tissue reconstruction technique. The graft is secured on the femoral side by looping through a soft tissue slit in the iliotibial band at the level of the lateral epicondyle. On the patellar side, slits are made within the proximal lateral patellar tendon and distal lateral quadriceps tendon. Passage of the graft recreates a V-shaped LPFL complex with its apex at the iliotibial band adjacent to the femoral origin of the LPFL (**Fig. 4**). Rehabilitation consists of an initial period of weight bearing as tolerated with a hinged knee brace locked in extension for 6 weeks. Full motion is

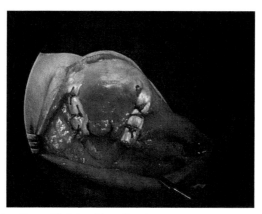

Fig. 4. LPFL reconstruction with lateral lengthening.

permitted when the patient is not bearing weight. Progressive strengthening begins at 6 weeks, with a goal of return to sport by 4 months.

Outcomes of Lateral Patellofemoral Ligament Reconstruction

There are limited data available on the outcomes of LPFL reconstruction owing to the rarity of the procedure and heterogeneity of techniques. One retrospective study of 19 reconstructions using an allograft LPFL reconstruction technique found significant improvements in Knee Injury and Osteoarthritis Outcome Scores after reconstruction.[60] In their cohort, Knee Injury and Osteoarthritis Outcome Scores improved from 34.39 preoperatively to 69.54 postoperatively at minimum of 2 years of follow-up. No patients reported residual medial patellar instability or apprehension. Another case series included 13 patients with iatrogenic medial instability who underwent iliotibial band–patellar tendon–based reconstruction as described elsewhere in this article.[63] At a minimum of 2 years of follow-up, Lysholm scores improved from 45.6 to 71.9, Western Ontario and McMaster Universities Osteoarthritis Index scores improved from 38 to 6, and mean patient satisfaction was rated at 8.2 out of 10.0 (range, 5–10). Sanchis-Alfonso reported 17 cases of LPFL reconstruction using an iliotibial band-based reconstruction technique with redirection of a central strip of iliotibial band to the lateral patella. At a minimum of 2 years of follow-up, visual analog scale scores improved from 7.6 to 1.9 and Lysholm scores improved from 36.4 to 86.1 with no recurrent medial patellar dislocations noted. Taken together, these limited reports do suggest that LPFL reconstruction is a viable and highly effective procedure regardless of differences in surgical technique.

SUMMARY

The LPFC is recognized as an important stabilizer to both medial and lateral displacement of the patella.[64] Soft tissue abnormalities of the LPFC can range from pathologic tightness to laxity, presenting with patellar instability, anterior knee pain, or arthritis. A clinical evaluation should be performed to confirm patellar dislocation, assess the integrity of the lateral and medial soft tissues, and explore the presence of other pathoanatomic factors that may need to be addressed. Lateral retinacular lengthening is recommended over lateral release owing to iatrogenic medial instability. A LPFL reconstruction can be performed to treat medial instability.

CLINICS CARE POINTS

- Patients with patellofemoral soft-tissue imbalance may present with a variety of symptoms, including pain, swelling, or overt lateral or medial dislocations. Diagnosis of medial instability can be aided by patellar bracing with improvement of symptoms or apprehension.

- In the setting of instability, comprehensive evaluation should include other underlying risk factors, such as trochlear dysplasia, malalignment, or patella alta, when considering surgical intervention.

- Presence of cartilage defects may necessitate a secondary procedure and therefore should be evaluated in conjunction with other pathology.

- Indications for lateral release have narrowed significantly due to concerns of iatrogenic medial instability. The favored technique is a lateral lengthening. An open approach is preferred to allow for a measured lateral lengthening that maintains the integrity of the joint capsule.

- In cases of medial instability, LPFL reconstruction is highly effective at restoring stability and improving symptoms, despite the heterogeneity in techniques.

REFERENCES

1. Jibri Z, Jamieson P, Rakhra KS, et al. Patellar maltracking: an update on the diagnosis and treatment strategies. Insights Imaging 2019;10:65.
2. Hinckel BB, Yanke AB, Lattermann C. When to Add Lateral Soft Tissue Balancing? Sports Med Arthrosc Rev 2019;27:e25–31.
3. Mazzola C, Mantovani D. Patellofemoral malalignment and chondral damage: current concepts. Joints 2013;1:27.
4. Manske RC, Davies GJ. Examination of the patellofemoral joint. Int J Sports Phys Ther 2016;11:831.
5. Hinckel BB, Arendt EA. Lateral retinaculum lengthening or release. Oper Tech Sports Med 2015;23:100–6.
6. Unal B, Hinckel BB, Sherman SL, et al. Comparison of lateral retinaculum release and lengthening in the treatment of patellofemoral disorders. Am J Orthop 2017; 46:224–8.
7. Diederichs G, Köhlitz T, Kornaropoulos E, et al. Magnetic Resonance Imaging Analysis of Rotational Alignment in Patients With Patellar Dislocations. Am J Sports Med 2012;41:51–7.
8. Colatruglio M, Flanigan DC, Harangody S, et al. Identifying Patients With Patella Alta and/or Severe Trochlear Dysplasia Through the Presence of Patellar Apprehension in Higher Degrees of Flexion. Orthop J Sports Med 2020;8. 2325967120925486.
9. Diederichs G, Issever AS, Scheffler S. MR Imaging of Patellar Instability: Injury Patterns and Assessment of Risk Factors. RadioGraphics 2010;30:961–81.
10. Endo Y, Shubin Stein BE, Potter HG. Radiologic assessment of patellofemoral pain in the athlete. Sports Health 2011;3:195–210.
11. Wilson PL, Black SR, Ellis HB, et al. Distal femoral valgus and recurrent traumatic patellar instability: is isolated varus producing distal femoral osteotomy a treatment option? J Pediatr Orthop 2018;38:e162–7.

12. Van Haver A, De Roo K, De Beule M, et al. The Effect of Trochlear Dysplasia on Patellofemoral Biomechanics: A Cadaveric Study With Simulated Trochlear Deformities. Am J Sports Med 2015;43:1354–61.
13. Heidenreich MJ, Camp CL, Dahm DL, et al. The contribution of the tibial tubercle to patellar instability: analysis of tibial tubercle–trochlear groove (TT-TG) and tibial tubercle–posterior cruciate ligament (TT-PCL) distances. Knee Surgery, Sports Traumatology,. Arthroscopy 2017;25:2347–51.
14. Camp CL, Heidenreich MJ, Dahm DL, et al. Individualizing the tibial tubercle–trochlear groove distance: patellar instability ratios that predict recurrent instability. Am J Sports Med 2016;44:393–9.
15. Mistovich RJ, Urwin JW, Fabricant PD, et al. Patellar tendon–lateral trochlear ridge distance: a novel measurement of patellofemoral instability. Am J Sports Med 2018;46:3400–6.
16. Loeb AE, Tanaka MJ. The medial patellofemoral complex. Curr Rev Musculoskelet Med 2018;11:201–8.
17. Shah KN, DeFroda SF, Ware JK, et al. Lateral patellofemoral ligament: An anatomic study. Orthop J Sports Med 2017;5. 2325967117741439.
18. DeFroda SF, Shah KN, Lemme N, et al. Biomechanical properties of the lateral patellofemoral ligament: A cadaveric analysis. Orthopedics 2018;41:e797–801.
19. Capkin S, Zeybek G, Ergur I, et al. An anatomic study of the lateral patellofemoral ligament. Acta Orthop Traumatol Turc 2017;51:73–6.
20. Fulkerson JP, Gossling HR. Anatomy of the knee joint lateral retinaculum. Clin Orthop Relat Res 1980;153:183–8.
21. KAPLAN EB. Some aspects of functional anatomy of the human knee joint. Clin Orthop Relat Res 1962;23:18–29.
22. Navarro MS, Beltrani Filho CA, Akita Junior J, et al. Relationship between the lateral patellofemoral ligament and the width of the lateral patellar facet. Acta Ortop Bras 2010;18(1):19–22. Available at: http://www.scielo.br/aob.2010.
23. Reider B, Marshall JL, Koslin B, et al. The anterior aspect of the knee joint. J Bone Joint Surg Am 1981;63:351–6.
24. Waligora AC, Johanson NA, Hirsch BE. Clinical anatomy of the quadriceps femoris and extensor apparatus of the knee. Clin Orthop Relat Res 2009;467:3297–306.
25. Vieira ELC, Vieira EÁ, Da Silva RT, et al. An anatomic study of the iliotibial tract. Arthroscopy 2007;23:269–74.
26. Yanke AB, Huddleston HP, Campbell K, et al. Effect of Patella Alta on the Native Anatomometricity of the Medial Patellofemoral Complex: A Cadaveric Study. Am J Sports Med 2020;48:1398–405.
27. Christian DR, Redondo ML, Cancienne JM, et al. Differential contributions of the quadriceps and patellar attachments of the proximal medial patellar restraints to resisting lateral patellar translation. Arthroscopy 2020;36:1670–6.
28. Merican AM, Kondo E, Amis AA. The effect on patellofemoral joint stability of selective cutting of lateral retinacular and capsular structures. J Biomech 2009;42:291–6.
29. Ghosh KM, Merican AM, Iranpour-Boroujeni F, et al. Length change patterns of the extensor retinaculum and the effect of total knee replacement. J Orthop Res 2009;27:865–70.
30. Pollard B, UNIVERSITY COLLEGE HOSPITAL. Old-standing (congenital) dislocation of patella ; reduction of patella after dividing the vastus externus and chiselling a new trochlear surface on the femur ; restoration of function of the limb. Lancet 1891;137:1203–4.

31. Schonholtz GJ, Zahn MG, Magee CM. Lateral retinacular release of the patella. Arthroscopy 1987;3:269–72.
32. Kolowich PA, Paulos LE, Rosenberg TD, et al. Lateral release of the patella: indications and contraindications. Am J Sports Med 1990;18:359–65.
33. Fu FH, Maday MG. Arthroscopic lateral release and the lateral patellar compression syndrome. Orthop Clin North Am 1992;23:601–12.
34. Ficat P, Ficat C, Bailleux A. [External hypertension syndrome of the patella. Its significance in the recognition of arthrosis]. Rev Chir Orthop Reparatrice Appar Mot 1975;61:39–59.
35. Stern SH, Moeckel BH, Insall JN. Total knee arthroplasty in valgus knees. Clin Orthop Relat Res 1991;5–8.
36. Lattermann C, Toth J, Bach BR Jr. The role of lateral retinacular release in the treatment of patellar instability. Sports Med Arthrosc Rev 2007;15:57–60.
37. Panni AS, Tartarone M, Patricola A, et al. Long-term results of lateral retinacular release. Arthroscopy 2005;21:526–31.
38. Nonweiler DE, DeLee JC. The diagnosis and treatment of medial subluxation of the patella after lateral retinacular release. Am J Sports Med 1994;22:680–6.
39. Liu JN, Steinhaus ME, Kalbian IL, et al. Patellar Instability Management: A Survey of the International Patellofemoral Study Group. Am J Sports Med 2018;46: 3299–306.
40. Merchant AC, Mercer RL. Lateral release of the patella. A preliminary report. Clin Orthop Relat Res 1974;40–5.
41. Miller GK, Dickason JM, Fox JM, et al. The use of electrosurgery for arthroscopic subcutaneous lateral release. Orthopedics 1982;5:309–14.
42. Fulkerson JP. Diagnosis and treatment of patients with patellofemoral pain. Am J Sports Med 2002;30:447–56.
43. Hallisey MJ, Doherty N, Bennett WF, et al. Anatomy of the junction of the vastus lateralis tendon and the patella. J Bone Joint Surg Am 1987;69:545–9.
44. Debell H, Pinter Z, Pinto M, et al. Vascular supply at risk during lateral release of the patella during total knee arthroplasty: A cadaveric study. J Clin Orthop Trauma 2019;10:107–10.
45. Hamawandi SA, Amin HI, Al-Humairi AK. Open versus arthroscopic release for lateral patellar compression syndrome: a randomized-controlled trial. Arch Orthop Trauma Surg 2021.
46. Larson RL, Cabaud HE, Slocum DB, et al. The patellar compression syndrome: surgical treatment by lateral retinacular release. Clin Orthop Relat Res 1978;158–67.
47. Slocum DB, Larson RL. Surgical Treatment of the Dislocating Patella in Athletes. Annual Meeting of the American Orthopaedic Association; 1973 June 28, 1973; Homestead, Hot Springs, Virginia.
48. Ceder LC, Larson RL. Z-plasty lateral retinacular release for the treatment of patellar compression syndrome. Clin Orthop Relat Res 1979;110–3.
49. Levy BJ, Jimenez AE, Fitzsimmons KP, et al. Medial patellofemoral ligament reconstruction and lateral retinacular lengthening in the skeletally immature patient. Arthrosc Tech 2020;9:e737–45.
50. Hinckel B, Arendt E. Lateral Retinaculum Lengthening/Release. Oper Tech Sports Med 2015;23.
51. Merican AM, Amis AA. Anatomy of the lateral retinaculum of the knee. J Bone Joint Surg Br Vol 2008;90-B:527–34.

52. Vogel LA, Pace JL. Trochleoplasty, medial patellofemoral ligament reconstruction, and open lateral lengthening for patellar instability in the setting of high-grade trochlear dysplasia. Arthrosc Tech 2019;8:e961–7.
53. O'Neill DB. Open lateral retinacular lengthening compared with arthroscopic release. A prospective, randomized outcome study. J Bone Joint Surg Am 1997;79:1759–69.
54. Pagenstert G, Wolf N, Bachmann M, et al. Open lateral patellar retinacular lengthening versus open retinacular release in lateral patellar hypercompression syndrome: a prospective double-blinded comparative study on complications and outcome. Arthroscopy 2012;28:788–97.
55. Merchant AC. Is it lateral retinacular lengthening versus lateral retinacular release or over-release? Arthroscopy 2013;29:403.
56. Teitge RA, Torga Spak R. Lateral patellofemoral ligament reconstruction. Arthroscopy 2004;20:998–1002.
57. Loeb AE, Farr J, Parikh SN, et al. Noniatrogenic Medial Patellar Dislocations: Case Series and International Patellofemoral Study Group Experience. Orthop J Sports Med 2021;9. 232596712098553.
58. Saper MG, Shneider DA. Lateral Patellofemoral Ligament Reconstruction Using a Quadriceps Tendon Graft. Arthrosc Tech 2014;3:e445–8.
59. Saper M. Lateral Patellofemoral Ligament Reconstruction With a Gracilis Allograft. Arthrosc Tech 2018;7:e405–10.
60. Beckert M, Crebs D, Nieto M, et al. Lateral patellofemoral ligament reconstruction to restore functional capacity in patients previously undergoing lateral retinacular release. World J Clin Cases 2016;4:202–6.
61. Sawyer GA, Cram T, LaPrade RF. Lateral patellotibial ligament reconstruction for medial patellar instability. Arthrosc Tech 2014;3:e547–50.
62. Hughston JC, Flandry F, Brinker MR, et al. Surgical correction of medial subluxation of the patella. Am J Sports Med 1996;24:486–91.
63. Moatshe G, Cram TR, Chahla J, et al. Medial patellar instability: treatment and outcomes. Orthop J Sports Med 2017;5. 2325967117699816.
64. Sanchís-Alfonso V, Montesinos-Berry E, Monllau J, et al. Results of Isolated Lateral Retinacular Reconstruction for Iatrogenic Medial Patellar Instability. Arthroscopy 2014;31.

Printed and bound by CPI Group (UK) Ltd, Croydon, CR0 4YY

08/05/2025

01864704-0005